NEED TO LOSE WEIGHT QUICKLY FOR A SPECIAL OCCASION? HAVING TROUBLE SHEDDING THOSE FIRST FEW POUNDS?

Find out 7 ways to jump-start any diet with these quick and effective strategies:

DISCOVER:

—a diet that will also help you cleanse and purify your body, getting rid of toxins that have built up over many years

—an especially fast way to slim down without cooking

—how to lose weight fast *and* cut down meal preparation by eating only one food for two days straight

—a simple soup diet that's loaded with fiber— and may even help prevent cancer

—an easy, delicious way to get your recommended seven servings of fruits and vegetables every day

—healthful ways to indulge in some of your favorite foods—hamburgers, fish, eggs and cheese— and still lose weight

—a nutritious meal plan that allows you to eat eight small meals a day, choosing from a wide variety of foods

All the information you need on a host of pound-shedding diets is here!

Including quick and easy recipes...daily menu planners im in g
tips on ess fr

D0594895

THE

7

Most Effective Ways to Jump-Start Your Diet

Carmel Berman Reingold

Foreword by
Gail Piazza, B.S., M.A.,
Foods and Nutrition

A Dell Book

Published by
Dell Publishing
a division of
Random House, Inc.
1540 Broadway
New York, New York 10036

ISBN: 0-440-22587-6

Printed in the United States of America

Published simultaneously in Canada

January 1999

10   9   8   7   6   5   4   3   2   1

WCD

As with all new dietary regimens, the jump-start diets described in this book should be followed only after first consulting with a physician. The author and publisher expressly disclaim responsibility for any adverse effects that may result from the use or application of the information contained in this book.

CONTENTS

Dieting is a major industry in this country. Not a week goes by that you don't see articles about losing weight in almost every magazine. But dieting alone has never been the real answer. Sure, you will lose a few pounds, but sooner or later you will gain them back. Doctors and nutritionists agree that this yo-yo dieting syndrome can cause health problems. So what is the answer? Lifestyle changes. Educating yourself about your own eating habits and proper nutrition is the first step. In fact, in order to make your weight loss permanent, you must first forget the words "I'm on a diet." Having a basic knowledge of nutrition and learning the fat and calorie content of the foods you eat is essential. Next, and possibly most important, is that you must be psychologically ready to make a long-term commitment to lifetime changes. To many people, food has become an addiction much the same as smoking. Only when you make this commitment to yourself will you be successful in taking off weight and keeping it off.

As a nutritionist, I am generally not in favor of crash diets, because they promote rapid weight loss but do nothing to address the real problems that have made a diet necessary. I do feel, however, that nothing helps you succeed like success. *The 7 Most Effective Ways to Jump-Start Your Diet* has been written to help you get yourself psychologically ready to lose weight permanently. This quick-fix success could be what prompts you to continue to get yourself in better shape. Pick the diet that appeals to you most and follow it closely. The reason why you need to lose weight quickly—perhaps to fit into a dress or suit, or to look good for that special occasion—is not really important. What is important is that when you have lost those initial pounds, you must take the time to reflect on your future health and well-being. Don't slip back into the same routine. This time, do yourself a favor and make the commitment to change your eating habits and the way you view food, and start some sort of fitness program. A healthful diet coupled with exercise is the only effective way to maintain proper weight.

In a previous book, *The Lifelong Anti-Cancer Diet*, Carmel Reingold interpreted the National Academy of Science's groundbreaking findings that helped to determine that the type of foods that we eat and omit from our diets are important in preventing cancer. She supplied menus, recipes, and general information that helped to demystify this weighty report. Now she addresses the problem of overeating, which also threatens good health. In *The 7 Most Effective Ways to Jump-Start Your Diet* she provides the information that can start you quickly on the road to better health.

So once you have jump-started your diet and are psyched because you look and feel better, where do you go? The government has revamped the basic four food groups and replaced them with the U.S. Department of Agriculture's Food Pyramid. The pyramid provides a basic lesson in how and what to eat. The foods at the base should comprise the bulk of what you should eat daily. As you move up on the pyramid, fewer servings of each food group are recommended, until you reach the top, which is the group with the fewest number of servings. The food group at the base consists of bread, cereal, rice, and pasta; the recommendation is for 6 to 11 servings per day. Moving up, the next group is vegetables (3 to 5 servings) and fruit (2 to 4 servings). Next is the protein group, consisting of 2 to 3 servings of dairy products and 2 to 3 servings of meats, poultry, fish, eggs, and nuts. The group at the very top of the pyramid is the fat group, consisting of fats, oils, and sugar; these are to be used sparingly.

Changing the amount and types of food on your plate will help establish better eating habits. Fill half the plate with vegetables and fruits, one-quarter with foods from the grain group, and the other quarter with foods from the protein groups. By increasing the amounts of whole grains, fruits, and vegetables that you eat, you increase the amount of fiber that you consume. In addition to being lower in fat and calories, fruits and vegetables are high in vitamins, minerals, beta carotene, and fiber. Making these changes is a move toward better health, because this type of diet helps to fight certain cancers and promote good heart health.

Don't become overwhelmed. If you have a plan, and you take things step by step, you will find that accomplishing these long-term goals isn't as difficult as it seems. The next step is to evaluate what you eat. Do so by keeping a journal for one week. Don't change your eating habits at all. Just write down everything that you eat, with the exact amounts. Start reading the nutritional information on food labels to see what a serving size is as well as the amount of calories and fat in that amount of food. A pocket calorie counter and a small diet scale also are good tools to help you learn the composition of common foods. Once you start weighing what you eat, you probably will discover that you eat much more than you think you do and that what you think is a serving is more like two. Note the time of day and mood you were in when you decided it was time to eat. You also might discover from your journal that many times you are eating out of boredom or frustration rather than hunger. That is where the exercise comes in. If you find that certain stresses or emotions trigger an eating binge, try doing some exercise at that time; if that isn't possible, do something you enjoy to lift your mood or get you away from the temptation to eat when you're not hungry. Remember to start exercising slowly. If you do too much, you will increase the risk of injury. Slowly increase your activity until you have reached the desired amount of exercise. Generally speaking, your goal should be 30 minutes a day, four or five times a week. Be sure to get your doctor's okay before you begin any exercise program.

Study your journal, and add up how many calories you eat in a day. Now that you have that all-important resolve, and you are ready to change the way you eat and the way you view food, it is time to reduce the amount of calories that you consume each day. The bottom line is that calories count. For every 3,500 calories you eat or don't eat, you will gain or lose a pound. A 2-pounds-a-week weight loss is desirable. Weight that is lost slowly is easier to keep off than weight lost quickly. Don't set unrealistic goals. Even if you want to lose 50 pounds, think small; set your sights on 10 pounds at a time. When you reach that goal, give yourself a *nonfood* reward. Don't make certain foods taboo. If you really crave a certain food, fit it into your allotted calories for the day or make up for it the next day. If you deny yourself everything you love, you will wind up compensating by eating more of something else, and you will still feel deprived. Remember, your goal is a long-term one.

By following these basic guidelines and, also, drinking plenty of water, getting enough sleep, and

Now You Can Jump-Start Your Diet

There just may be one person in a million who hasn't yearned to lose weight at one time or another. We are a society concerned about being overweight, dieting, and body image. In fact, dieting, for many, is a way of life, and marching right alongside is the concomitant complaint: "I've tried dieting and it just doesn't work for me." Sound familiar? If you're reading this book then probably you've said that more than once. Likely you may have consulted nutritionists, diet centers, doctors, books, or followed the advice in your favorite magazine. You have understood—and agreed—that a sensible diet, one that works to change bad eating habits, is the best way to go. You've dutifully done all the right things: Perhaps you've counted calories, or maybe you've added up fat grams, or possibly you've measured portions, followed a point system, balanced protein against carbohydrates, or traded a favorite sweet for a plateful of pasta. There seem to be as many ways of dieting as there are stars in the sky—but yet none of them seems to work for you.

Or you may grudgingly admit that those good-little-girl diets do work, but at what feels like an excruciatingly slow pace, perhaps taking off one or maybe two pounds each week. No doubt that after a few weeks of feeling denied and unloved (we know food is love), you give up and go back to eating the foods you enjoy, saying to yourself, "Forget it! Diets just don't work for me."

This is especially true if, after two or three weeks of dieting, you look into that unfriendly mirror and see no change. And if that mirror isn't evil enough, there are those skinny jeans that have been hanging in your closet for months—the ones that were on sale and can't be returned. They didn't exactly fit when you bought them, but you were sure that after that diet which assigns points to every food item they would look just great on you. May as well give them away, right? You hate to see them every time you open the closet door since they're a constant reminder of your failure to lose weight.

Diets That Work . . . and Work Fast

If that scenario sounds familiar, here are two things you should do:

1. Don't give up on the jeans.
2. Try one of the marvelously effective short-term programs from this book that can jump-start your diet!

We are not talking here about diets to follow for many weeks or months. Many of these diets require a commitment of only a few days and should not be followed beyond the recommended time. They are intended to give your long-range dieting plans a jump-start—something a sensible weight-loss program often needs. The quick results these diets offer prove that you can lose weight. Instead of losing two pounds in two weeks, you just may lose five pounds in two days!

You will finally believe that your bathroom scale isn't broken, and that the numbers can move down as well as up.

Special Weight-Loss Needs

There may be other reasons why you want to jump-start your diet. Maybe you're going to a beach resort, and you want to wear a bathing suit cut up to here and down to there, or perhaps you're a member of a wedding party and you want to look almost as good as the bride when you walk down the aisle. If it's not a job interview, vacation, or wedding, your plans may include a very special party. Whatever the event, you know that losing weight is crucial to your confidence and ultimately your happiness. Of course, some people might not call these "good" reasons to follow a quick diet plan—but they are not in your shoes or your mind, and they are not aware of how far a little weight loss can go to boost your self-confidence, mental health, and self-esteem. It is important to understand and remember that none of these jump-start plans should be followed for a long time. We are talking about short-term dieting that can answer immediate needs and provide the incentive for you to start a slow—but healthful—diet plan.

Talking to Your Doctor

While many doctors would say that it's not healthy to lose weight too fast, you should realize that these jump-start diets last only for a few days. It's unlikely you can hurt yourself by lowering your caloric intake for a short time unless you have a medical condition that requires a certain diet. Certainly any of these diets is better than bingeing or starving yourself.

Before you embark on any of the following jump-start diets, you *must* talk to your doctor. Be honest with him or her and with yourself. Explain why you want to lose weight quickly. This is the moment for revelation and plain speaking. There's nothing shameful about your need to lose weight.

"I went to a shrink for a year," said Annabelle, a

stockbroker, "but I was afraid I'd sound like a bimbo if I told him how important losing weight was to my psyche. It took me a long time to admit to him—and to me—that a slim body is a top priority to me."

Looking good and feeling good about your appearance is not a frivolous desire. When you talk to your doctor, mention which of the jump-start diets you are considering, and then let him or her tell you if this diet is safe for you. *Don't start any diet without checking with your doctor first.*

The Temptation of Dieting

Maybe you never thought you'd be tempted to stay on a diet, but one that takes off pounds quickly can be very seductive. As you lose two or five or ten or even more pounds in days rather than months, you might be tempted to stay on one of the diets that follow beyond the number of days suggested.

Don't do it! Jump-start diets are intended to be of short duration. They don't offer the complete nutrition that you need for good health. Use a jump-start diet as an inspiring beginning—a time of instant gratification that will act as an incentive for a long-term plan that will take off pounds slowly and safely.

Motivation

"I kept telling myself that I wanted to lose weight," said Jeanine, 25, a nurse, "but did I really? I was a secret snacker. When no one was around I'd eat constantly—cookies, potato chips, ice cream—whatever was around. It took me a long time to admit that I didn't really want to lose weight—those extra pounds protected me from becoming involved in the dating game. Who needs guys, anyway? Besides, if someone really loved me, he'd love me fat or thin. Yeah, right. Except that before someone got to know me, he'd have to get past the fact that I was fat. Sure, I was a beautiful person within—but who knew about all that inner beauty? Once I faced the reality that looks *do* count, I was able to jump-start my diet. With a five-day plan during which I ate nothing but protein, I went down from 150 pounds to 140 pounds. I'm a little over five foot two, so those 10 pounds really made a difference. After that, I went on a plan where I lost a pound a week. I'm down a total of 20 pounds and I feel good about myself."

How Much Weight Will I Lose?

The amount of weight you will lose depends on the basic *you:* how much weight you need to lose; your metabolism, level of activity, bone structure, occupation; and, most important, your ability to stay on the jump-start diet of your choice. Yes, one cookie does count, as does just one tiny teaspoon of ice cream. Because jump-start diets are of such short duration, *any* cheating will make them ineffective.

Some jump-start dieters lose two pounds in two days, others lose five, still others find that eight unnecessary pounds have slipped away. Fasts—see the water fast and the juice diets—work more quickly than others.

While Dieting . . .

Don't cheat by eating some little thing that's not on the diet. A candy bar can make all your efforts worthless, as can skipping one of the recommended meals or substituting an inappropriate food. Do that, and the entire plan unravels. One skipped meal can make you inordinately hungry, and that can undermine the entire diet.

Should You Supplement Your Jump-Start Diet?

Many doctors say that if you eat well-balanced meals, you don't need to take supplements. Many of the jump-start diets are not well balanced but, as mentioned, they are intended to be followed only for a short time. Should you take a supplement while jump-starting your diet?

Here again, we must send you off to talk to your doctor. Some physicians recommend vitamins, especially C and E, whether you are on a diet or not. Possibly, your doctor might suggest a multivitamin while you are dieting or may recommend an increase of supplements you currently are taking. However, it's important to remember that the directions on many supplements recommend that the supplements be taken with food. Therefore, you need to be extra careful about what you ingest when you are following the water or liquid diets.

We can't give a blanket answer regarding the pros and cons of dietary supplements for all who follow a jump-start diet. Your health, the medications you may be taking, and the opinion of a doctor you trust must all be weighed before you can make an intelligent decision as to supplements.

Times When You Shouldn't Diet

- *You're going on vacation.* There you are, getting on and off planes, taking a cruise, staying at hotels, eating on the road. An impossible time to start on a diet.

- *You've just given up smoking.* That's wonderful and *stressful. . . .* It's hard to give up nicotine and food at the same time. Unfortunately, many people who stop smoking often substitute food for cigarettes. Try tea or a diet soda when you feel you must have something. And go on a jump-start diet after you've conquered the craving for cigarettes.

- *You're facing an important business decision.* You need to concentrate on work, not on dieting.

- *You've invited someone really important to dinner.* You can't be the dieter at your own table when you've prepared (or bought at the local caterer) a fabulous three-course meal.

- *There's a family emergency,* such as illness or a hospital stay by someone close to you. With a lot to cope with, you have a valid excuse to postpone a jump-start diet.

- *You are very thin.* If your mother, your friends, and

especially your doctor tell you that you are already too thin, *do not* go on a jump-start diet. Anorexia is as unsightly as obesity, and bingeing can be more dangerous than overeating. If you're having a problem seeing yourself as the thin person you really are, it may be time to consult a therapist.

Choosing the Diet That's Right for You

You've checked with your doctor, looked into your soul, did one final check in the mirror, and you've decided to go on a jump-start diet. Now the only decision you have to make is to choose the diet that's right for you. Here are some considerations:

A jump-start diet is not meant to create stress but rather to relieve the despondency you experience when you get on a scale, look into a mirror, or try on slim jeans. You know yourself better than anyone: what you like to eat, how much tolerance you have, what your schedule is like, and what your body needs. Based on all that, you should be able to figure out which of the jump-start diets is right for you at this time. You are being offered a lot of choices, and you probably will find more than one diet appealing, but not every diet is right for everyone.

For example, included here is a water fast and diets that are based on liquid meals. Could you limit your intake for 24 or 48 hours to water or juice? If you are thinking "No way, no how," you know these diets are not right for you. However, if it's summer and you can't seem to get enough of melons, berries, and other luscious fruits, take advantage of a "fruit only" weekend.

The second main purpose of a jump-start diet—the first obviously is to lose weight—is to make you feel good about yourself. If you start out by thinking that a diet will be impossible for you to follow, then it probably will be. Don't embark on a jump-start diet if just thinking about it makes you shake with negative vibes. Do that, and you're programming yourself for failure.

Before you start on any of these diets, read about them. More than one diet will be appealing and seem doable for a short time. For example, if hamburgers and steak are some of your favorite foods, try the Argentine Diet, which comes to you from that beef-loving country. However, if you wrinkle your nose at the idea of meat and love all kinds of fish and shellfish, the Think-Fish Diet will be easy to follow. And monodieting may be just the thing for those who love starchy foods. Choose the diet or diets that you find most appealing and in sync with your tastes and lifestyle. We've divided the diets into seven programs with a little something for everyone. They are:

1. The 1- or 2-Day Water Fast
2. The Whole-Foods Method with Fruits and Vegetables
3. The Liquid Way
4. The Protein Approach
5. Cabbage Soup and Other Souper Diets
6. 3-Day Smart Grazing plan
7. 1- or 2-Day Monodiet

Psychologically Speaking

Before you embark on a jump-start, or any other, diet, prepare your mind as well as your body. Plan ahead. Most people start dieting on a Friday or Monday—choose the day that fits your schedule, and mark it as Day 1 on your calendar three days in advance.

During those three days allow your imagination to roam. Stretch out on the couch, close your eyes, and picture yourself pounds thinner. Wow! You look so good. Think of that long, clingy skirt you've been eyeing for weeks. Can't you see yourself going into that boutique, trying it on, and having it fit! You'll buy it and wear it to that new club you've been dying to go to.

Dieting is much easier if you plan ahead and pursue other activities. Rather than concentrating on what you will or will not eat, plan on going to a museum. How about joining a gym, or learning to play tennis? Go anywhere *except* to your favorite restaurant—that's no place to pursue a jump-start diet.

And After Dieting . . .

You've completed your jump-start diet, and the results make you really happy. You've lost enough weight to indicate how really good you can look, and you're proud of yourself for having maintained the required discipline of the diet. You deserve a reward! Sure you do, and let that reward be those ankle boots you've longed for, or those big hoop earrings—

anything but food. This is the moment to face the influence that food has had in your life: When depressed you looked to a candy bar for comfort; when successful at an endeavor you felt you deserved chocolate cake. But this is the first day of the new, thinner you, and now you can face up to the real definition of food: Food is not comfort, not a reward, not love. Food provides nourishment for the body. Think of food that way rather than as the all-healing ingredient for problems of the heart, mind, psyche, and soul.

And remember, too, that you can put the weight back on just as easily as you took it off if you return to the eating habits that caused you to gain weight in the first place. This is the pivotal moment to move on to a smart diet—which offers nutrition with reduced calorie and fat content. This doesn't mean that you have to get out a gram scale and measure every bite, nor does it mean that you have to count calories. If you've dieted before—and who hasn't?—you know that ice cream contains more fat than an apple and that chicken or fish contains less fat than a marbled steak. Relax. A less rigid approach to what you eat is the only way you can continue on a long-term weight-loss plan.

DIET DOS AND DON'TS

- *Do* walk as much as often as possible. Don't take a bus or a car if you can comfortably walk the same distance.

- *Don't* binge the day before you start dieting. That makes dieting that much harder.

- *Do* ease into a diet by eating slightly less for two or three days before you start on the diet.

- *Do* decide what you're going to eat before you go to a restaurant, and if you go off your diet for a day or a meal, don't give up. Go back jump-starting the next day.

- If you're going on a 10-Day Jump-Start Diet, don't worry about how you'll get through the next 10 days. *Do* it one day at a time.

- *Do* make yourself as happy and as comfortable as you can while dieting. Don't eat a diet meal standing by the microwave. Do set a table— even if it's just for you—with your prettiest dishes and a stemmed glass to hold sparkling water.

- *Do* try to exercise and keep active while dieting. Go places where you can't eat, such as a museum or the ballet.

- *Don't* give in to the "just one" temptation—as in "I'll have just one cookie." The ad campaign that said "I bet you can't eat just one" was absolutely on the money.

- *Do* drink lots of water—unless you're on the water fast. Water is filling and rids the body of toxins.

- *Do* make dry brushing a daily habit. Using a body brush or a loofah, brush your body all over as a way of ridding your body of the toxins that rise to the surface as you diet. Remember, your skin, like your kidneys, is an organ of elimination. Dry brushing not only will enhance circulation but will help get rid of dead skin cells.

1

The 1- or 2-Day Water Fast

For over ten years I would take a weekend every few months and go on a water fast. For 35 to 48 hours I would drink only purified water. When the weekend was over, I felt cleansed, energized, and all my congestive problems would clear up. Food and everything else tasted so much better afterward—and, of course, there was a bonus of dropping a few pounds in the process.

—Judy, 45, writer

Doctors and nutritionists are divided when it comes to a water fast in which nothing is taken but water for one or two days. Dr. Andrew Weil, in his book *Spontaneous Healing,* has written that "At different times in my life I have experimented with fasting one day a week. . . . When I fast I consume nothing but water or herb tea . . . and I find this to be a useful physical and psychological discipline. It feels healthy."

Dr. Weil does say, however, that no one who is sensitive to cold or who is already quite thin should pursue a water fast.

On the other hand, holistic health practitioners Shoshanna Katzman and Wendy Shankin-Cohen, authors of *Feeling Light: The Holistic Solution to Permanent Weight Loss and Wellness*, recommend a water fast, because they believe that such a fast can "undo the effects of years of toxic buildup." They explain that too much food overloads the system and is not properly digested. And it is this undigested food that accumulates in our bodies and turns into excess fat.

Be aware that a number of nutritionists believe that a water fast is too hard on the body; they prefer a fasting program built around a variety of juices.

If You Decide to Go on a Water Fast

Check this and all other diets out with your doctor. If you have any medical problems, this fast may not be for you.

Before you begin, ask yourself: "How do I really feel about having nothing but water for 24 to 48 hours?" Does it sound almost frighteningly difficult? If so, the water fast is not the jump-start diet for you. If, however, this experience seems purifying and cleansing, you may be ready for a water fast.

To Prepare

It's best to ease into a water fast. Try this fast on a weekend when you don't need those calories for work, and when you're not surrounded by friends or colleagues who ask you what time you want to have lunch or go for drinks after work. If you schedule your water fast for the weekend, start eating lightly on Thursday and Friday. Have tea with or without lemon for breakfast and toasted whole-grain bread. Lunch should be a salad or a clear soup. For dinner, have cooked vegetables with rice or a small steamed or baked potato. Keep food shopping to a minimum before the fast, and toss out all food that might be a temptation: good-bye, cookies; farewell, potato chips.

The Water Fast

You will have only water and tea—any kind—for the next 24 or 48 hours. Some nutritionists who advocate a water fast recommend drinking distilled or mineral water. Perhaps you would enjoy a variety of imported bottled water. You may use a lemon wedge with the water and the tea, and you can drink as much water or tea as you wish.

Instead of thinking of this fast as something difficult you must get through, imagine that you're staying at an expensive spa. Drink water from your very best goblets, and pamper yourself with a facial or a manicure and a pedicure. Give in to that urge to buy all the magazines that you want. This light diet goes best with light reading.

Should you continue with this fast for a second day? That depends on how you feel when you wake up the next morning. If you feel weak, exceptionally fatigued, or mentally depressed, don't go on with the fast. If you feel healthier, somehow, and psychologically better for being so disciplined, you may continue the water fast for a second day.

After the Fast

A stringent fast requires a slow return to regular meals. Have sliced fresh fruit for the first two meals followed by broth and tea; or have tea and toast for breakfast followed by clear broth with crackers or toast for lunch. Dinner can be vegetable soup or chicken-noodle soup with crackers or toast.

Sharon, 35, who goes on a 2-Day Water Fast every six months, says that when she goes off the fast she has tea and toast for breakfast, vegetable-noodle soup for lunch, and a small piece of broiled fish or chicken with a cooked vegetable for dinner.

"Having had nothing but water and tea for two days really cuts down on my appetite. After a water fast, a small portion of simple foods taste absolutely delicious. The last time I went on a water fast I lost seven pounds in two days—that made me feel really good about myself."

2

The Whole-Foods Method with Fruits and Vegetables

My brother made fun of me when I was a kid, because my idea of a great snack was a carrot, celery stalk, or apple, but my father told me to ignore my brother and said I was doing the right thing. As I grew older, I got away from munching raw vegetables and fruit, and I kept a package of cookies in my bottom desk drawer. Well, you can imagine what happened. Now when I want to lose five or ten pounds I go back to my good, childhood habits and I brown-bag veggies or fresh fruit to the office. It works! Last month I lost five pounds in three days by eating raw vegetables.

—Susan, 38, librarian

If it wasn't your mother, it probably was your grand-mother who told you to eat your fruits and vegetables for all those vitamins and minerals. Despite that good advice—and all of us like to ignore good advice most of the time—you may have grown up liking fruits and vegetables. If that's so, we have a great way for you to jump-start your diet. Actually, we have six ways, all based on three days of eating mainly fruits and vegetables.

Why is produce a dieter's delight? Because vegetables are low in calories. While fruit, because of its sugar content, is higher in calories than veggies, the calorie count is still low when compared to most other foods. Some fruits and vegetables contain a trace of fat, but that's certainly offset by the fiber content, which makes you feel full and want to eat less. Fiber also is believed to lower those "bad" cholesterol numbers, and many fruits and vegetables contain nutrients that are said to lower the risk of some cancers.

Are You Clean or Dirty Inside?

A current buzz word, heard a great deal in holistic and new age circles, is "cleansing." Those who use that word imply that intestinally we are all dirty, and our insides must be cleaned out from time to time for optimum health. (About 75 years ago this same theory was popular, and in those days castor oil, enemas, and lots of bran were recommended as the way to go.)

Dr. Andrew Weill says that fasting or low-fat, low-calorie diets give the digestive system a rest, and that's how we look at it. You may feel cleansed and lighter after eating produce for three days, but it's not necessary to imply that you were ever dirty in the first place.

Raw vs. Cooked Produce

Only one of the following jump-start methods uses cooked vegetables. According to one holistic theory, raw fruits and vegetables are especially effective when trying to lose weight, because they are loaded with enzymes. Says Deborah Mitchell in *Natural Medicine for Weight Loss*, "Enzymes help convert foods into nutrients the body can use in order to digest food and initiate metabolic activity. Enzyme deficiencies can cause insufficient absorption of food and food cravings." A shortage of enzymes, some believe, causes food to turn into fat. The whole-foods program includes diets of raw fruits and vegetables—no vitamins or minerals lost in cooking—as well as one diet of cooked vegetables.

These Diets Sound Easy, So . . .

No, don't stay on any of these diets for longer than three days. Because these diets lack high protein, they do not offer all the nutrients you need for good health. Any long-term diet without protein means that the weight you lose will be muscle, and that's not a healthy way to go. Before you try any of these low-protein diets, talk to your doctor.

3-DAY CITRUS FRUIT DIET

Before you start, stock up on as many different kinds of citrus fruit as you can find. Grapefruit comes in white, pink, and ruby red. From the family of oranges you can choose navels, mineolas, clementines, temples, and blood oranges. Buy some tangelos, tangerines, and, if you can find it, ugli fruit from the Caribbean. Ugli fruit is a cross between a grapefruit and an orange and has a bumpy skin. It is well named.

For the next three days you can eat as much citrus fruit as you wish. Beverages include water and all flavors of diet soda, including the sparkling waters that contain fruit flavors but no sugar. Coffee and tea are allowed, and you can have a sugar substitute, but no milk in your coffee. If you like, you can sprinkle sugar substitute on the grapefruit.

The following is a sample menu. Stay on it for three days *only*, switching citrus fruits around as you wish.

ALL BREAKFASTS
  Grapefruit
  1 slice whole-grain bread, or ½ bagel, or 1 whole-
    wheat roll
  Coffee or tea

MIDMORNING SNACKS
  Tangerines or tangelos

ALL LUNCHES
  Nonfat beef broth or chicken broth
  An assortment of oranges
  Diet soda

ALL AFTERNOON SNACKS
  Ugli fruit or tangerines
  2 slices American cheese
  2 whole-grain crackers
  Iced tea

ALL DINNERS
  Fruit salad made of segments of assorted citrus fruits
    with 2 tablespoons any fat-free salad dressing
  Sparkling water (may be fruit flavored if noncaloric)

3-DAY GRAPEFRUIT AND COTTAGE CHEESE DIET

Grapefruit and cottage cheese are a good combination. The tart grapefruit nicely complements the tangy, slightly creamy cottage cheese. You can have as much grapefruit as you wish—and we recommend buying as many different kinds as you can find. As for the cottage cheese, you can have 4 cups of the creamy, or 4 percent fat, cottage cheese, or 6 cups of the light, low-fat, or pot-style cottage cheese.

  The following is a sample menu. Do not stay on this diet for longer than three days.

ALL BREAKFASTS
  Grapefruit
  Cottage cheese
  1 slice whole-grain bread, toasted
  Coffee or tea with artificial sweetener

MIDMORNING SNACKS
  Grapefruit

ALL LUNCHES
  Nonfat beef broth or chicken broth
  Grapefruit
  Cottage cheese
  Diet soda

ALL DINNERS
  Grapefruit segments and cottage cheese on a bed of
    shredded lettuce with 2 tablespoons any fat-free
    salad dressing
  2 whole-grain crackers
  Sparkling water (may be fruit flavored if noncaloric)

3-DAY FRENCH CRUDITÉS DIET

Crudités—French for an assortment of raw vegetables—are a great, munchable, crunchable way to lose weight. The bulk and fiber provided by the raw veggies lessens hunger pangs—especially when you know you're allowed to eat as many of them as you wish. This 3-day program also includes dips and dressings that will add flavor, spice, and color to meals. For beverages you may have water, tea or coffee, with artificial sweetener, and skim milk. Diet sodas are allowed, including our favorites—fruit-flavored sparkling waters that contain no calories. Repeat the following menu for three days.

ALL BREAKFASTS
1 whole-wheat roll or 2 slices whole-grain bread
Coffee or tea (with skim milk, optional)

ALL LUNCHES AND DINNERS
As much as you want of the following raw vegetables: green, red, yellow and brown bell peppers, broccoli sprouts, cabbage (shredded), carrot sticks, cauliflower florets, celery sticks, cherry tomatoes, cucumbers, endive, lettuce (all types), snow peas, radish (all types), scallions, spinach, sugar snap peas

Any fat-free salad dressing, or use one of the recipes for dressings or dips that follow

Iced tea or coffee

Any diet soda, including sparkling water (may be fruit flavored if noncaloric)

CREAMY HERB DRESSING

4 tablespoons nonfat sour cream
$\frac{1}{2}$ cup skim milk
1 small shallot, minced
1 scallion, finely chopped
1 tablespoon fresh cilantro, finely chopped
Salt and freshly ground pepper to taste

1. Combine sour cream and milk in a bowl. Mix until blended.
2. Stir in all remaining ingredients, and mix until combined.

Yield: About 1 cup

SPICY TOMATO DRESSING

1 cup tomato juice
1 tablespoon olive oil
1 tablespoon chopped flat or Italian parsley
1/4 teaspoon crushed red pepper flakes (or to taste)
Salt to taste

Combine all ingredients in a screw-top jar and shake until thoroughly blended.

Yield: About 1 cup

YOGURT-CUCUMBER DIP

1 cup plain, nonfat yogurt
1 medium cucumber, shredded
1 garlic clove, pressed
Salt and freshly ground pepper to taste
Fresh dill, chopped

1. Place yogurt in cheesecloth or in a colander lined with a cloth napkin. Allow water to drain overnight.
2. Using either your hands or a strainer, squeeze water out of shredded cucumbers.
3. Combine all ingredients in a bowl. Mix until thoroughly blended.

Yield: About 1½ cups

ORANGE DRESSING

1 cup orange juice
1 tablespoon olive oil
$1/4$ teaspoon hot pepper sauce (or to taste)
Salt and freshly ground pepper to taste

Combine all ingredients in a screw-top jar and shake until thoroughly blended.

Yield: About 1 cup

3-DAY VEGGIES-ALL-THE-WAY DIET

If you love vegetables and prefer them cooked rather than raw, this three-day diet may be the right one for you. All vegetables are allowed except for legumes, corn, and potatoes, and vegetables can be prepared your favorite way: stir-fried, roasted, even sautéed in a bit of olive oil. (See our recipe suggestions.) The only sauces you're not allowed are those prepared with butter or cream. Lunches and dinners can be a large serving of one of your favorite vegetables, or you can combine as many different vegetables as you like at one meal. Repeat the following menu for three days.

ALL BREAKFASTS

Low-fat cottage cheese

Coffee or tea (with artificial sweetener and skim milk, optional)

ALL LUNCHES AND DINNERS

As much of any and all vegetables (except for potatoes, corn, and legumes) cooked without butter or cream

1 slice whole-grain bread at lunch and at dinner

Any diet soda, including noncaloric fruit-flavored sparkling water

Tea or coffee, hot or iced

STIR-FRIED VEGETABLES

$\frac{1}{2}$ tablespoon olive oil
1 cup broccoli florets, steamed
10 asparagus spears, trimmed, cut in half
$\frac{1}{2}$ pound snow peas
$\frac{1}{4}$ cup nonfat chicken broth
1 tablespoon light soy sauce
1 teaspoon hot pepper sauce (optional)
Salt and freshly ground pepper to taste

1. Heat oil in a large, nonstick skillet. Add broccoli and asparagus and cook, stirring, until almost tender.
2. Add snow peas, broth, soy sauce, and hot pepper sauce.
3. Continue cooking, stirring, until all ingredients are cooked and heated through. Season to taste.

Serves: 2

QUICK SAUTÉ OF VEGETABLES

½ tablespoon olive oil
4 small zucchini, cut into 1-inch slices
2 red bell peppers, thinly sliced
4 plum tomatoes, quartered
1 small Spanish onion, thinly sliced
Salt and freshly ground pepper to taste

1. Heat oil in a large, nonstick skillet.
2. Add all vegetables, and sauté until heated and cooked through.
3. Season to taste.

Serves: 2

VEGETABLES ROASTED WITH OLIVE OIL AND LEMON

8 baby carrots
4 zucchini, cut into 2-inch slices
1 medium onion, quartered
2 red bell peppers, cut into large slices
2 cloves elephant garlic, sliced, or 1 garlic clove,
  minced
Salt and freshly ground pepper to taste
1 tablespoon olive oil
2 tablespoons lemon juice

1. Preheat oven to 375 degrees. Place all vegetables in a shallow, nonstick baking pan. Season to taste.
2. Combine oil and lemon in a screw-top jar. Shake until blended. Spoon mixture over vegetables.
3. Bake for 20 to 30 minutes, or until vegetables are crisp-tender.

Serves: 2

GREEN BEANS WITH SPICY TOMATO AND CARROT

1 pound green beans (not legumes) trimmed
1/2 tablespoon olive oil
4 plum tomatoes, coarsely chopped
1 small carrot, thinly sliced
1/4 teaspoon crushed red pepper flakes, or to taste
Salt to taste

1. Bring 1 quart water to boil. Add green beans and cook until just tender, about 15 minutes. Drain and rinse under cold, running water.
2. Heat oil in a nonstick skillet. Add beans, tomatoes, carrot, and red pepper flakes. Stir to combine. Cook, stirring occasionally, until tomatoes have dissolved and carrot is cooked. Season to taste.

Serves: 2

3-DAY SUMMER FRUIT DIET

"Summertime, and the living is easy . . ." was a line from one of the wonderful songs in George Gershwin's *Porgy and Bess*. The opening scene of the opera shows a street vendor selling fresh strawberries. A memorable moment—just as the fruits of summer are memorable. Sweet, succulent, full of flavor and color. July and August are the perfect months to go on a three-day diet of fresh fruits. The choices are many—and all yours. You can have a day of peaches and cherries, a day of melons, and a day of assorted berries. Or you can mix and match the fruits to suit your taste and daily whims. There are no recipes offered for the 3-Day Summer Fruit Diet, because summer's fresh fruits are best eaten raw. If you wish, you can add a dollop of plain, nonfat yogurt to a brimming soup plate of berries, sliced peaches or nectarines, but no other dressing is necessary.

ALL BREAKFASTS
   Cottage cheese (low-fat) or farmer's cheese
   1 whole-wheat roll, 1 slice whole-grain bread, or ½ bagel
   Coffee or tea (with artificial sweetener and skim milk, optional)

ALL LUNCHES AND DINNERS
   All the fresh fruit you want
   Plain nonfat yogurt (optional)
   Any diet soda, including fruit-flavored sparkling water (noncaloric) and plain water
   Tea or coffee, hot or iced

3

The Liquid Way

The juice diet is a little difficult for me, but after work I make myself a special cocktail which consists of juicing one pear, one apple, and a bit of ginger. I pour it over ice and squeeze some lemon on top. That relaxes and revitalizes me and usually does away with my desire for dinner. I lose several pounds that way when I have my "after-work special" for a few days in a row.
—Christina, 30, secretary

JUICE DIETS: HOW AND WHY THEY WORK

"First they talked about the four food groups," said Maida, "but that nutritional idea went out of style. Now they say you should eat a total of seven portions of fruits and vegetables each day! Well, I'm here to tell you that my day just isn't long enough!"

They. Who are the mysterious *they* telling us what to do? In this case *they* are nutritionists, dietitians, doctors concerned with health—all advising seven total servings of fruits and vegetables each day. Sounds like a lot? Let's see. If you have a small salad at lunch, followed by an apple, green beans plus a potato at night with an apple for dessert—that's still only five servings. And what about those days when you don't feel like eating a salad and would rather have a tuna sandwich? And it's hard to keep track.

But the good news is that, with juice, it's easy to have seven servings of fruits and vegetables—easy, delicious, and varied. And best of all, juices are the basis of a delicious jump-start diet.

What's in Juice?

You know that fruits and vegetables contain little or no fat and are loaded with vitamins and minerals—at least they start out that way. Once vegetables are cooked, however, much of that good stuff is dissipated and goes down the drain with water used for cooking.

And that's not all. Many vegetable dishes found in restaurants or fast-food takeouts are prepared with sauces, dressings, butter, or oil. The vegetables taste good, but the added fat doesn't help if you're trying to lose weight. You have a better chance with fresh fruit—as long as the fruit is eaten raw and not dipped in sugar or used as a base for a mousse or as a topping for an ice cream sundae.

How can you enjoy fruits and vegetables in their pristine state, with all their nutrients left intact? Eat them raw. But while fresh strawberries are enjoyable, fresh broccoli is not. Therefore, one of the best ways to retain the benefits of fruits and vegetables is to turn them into a variety of juices that can work really fast to take off pounds.

Juices containing nutrients and antioxidants (beta carotene, vitamins E and C), say nutritionists, can flush toxins out of your body, while juices prepared from cruciferous vegetables, such as cabbage, broccoli, and brussels sprouts, can help prevent certain types of cancer.

If You Decide to Jump-Start with Juice

If you don't already own a juicer, you may want to buy one. Currently two types of juicers are available: those that prepare juice from citrus fruits and heavy-duty machines that can be used for citrus fruits and for raw vegetables.

However, before you purchase a juicer, consider this: Most juices can be prepared successfully in a blender. Also, many food processors come with juicer attachments. Check out the appliances you already own if you don't want the expense of purchasing a juicer.

If you do use a blender or a food processor, you may have to add a small amount of water to prepare the juice, and the result may be a somewhat thicker beverage than one prepared with a heavy-duty juicer. However, you can strain the juice before drinking, if you wish.

Ready-Prepared Juices

Many supermarkets and specialty food shops offer an assortment of juices that are sugar and additive free. You may find the juices that you want there. You also can use frozen fruit juices—without added sugar—in your juice diet.

Be aware that recently there have been problems with nonpasteurized apple juice. Even though pasteurizing may kill some nutrients, it is safer to drink pasteurized juice.

While additive-free fruit juices are available, juices prepared from fresh vegetables are not—this is why you need a juicer, other appliance or a neighborhood juice bar that offers an array of freshly prepared vegetable juices. Could you follow a juice diet with nothing but fruit juices? You could, but a juice diet should contain both fruit and vegetable juices for more balance.

Before You Go on a Juice Diet

- Talk to your doctor first. If you have any medical problems, such as diabetes or hypoglycemia, a juice diet may not be right for you. No one under 17 years of age should try any of these diets, although fruit and vegetable juices can be a fine way to supplement a teenager's meal plan and an easy way to add nutrients to meals that seem to consist mainly of junk food.
- Follow the juice diet for three days—and only three days. If you wish, you can repeat this diet every three months—that is, of course, if your doctor gives you the okay.

- Ease into a juice diet by eating lightly the day before you start juicing. A breakfast of juice, followed by either coffee or tea and whole-grain toast or a toasted English muffin, is a good way to start. Lunch can be a favorite salad with chicken, salmon, or tuna; a dinner of broiled chicken or fish with a steamed vegetable and a baked potato is a good way to segue into a juice diet. Dessert or a snack after lunch and dinner can be any fresh fruit. Wake up the next morning, and you're ready to begin your juice diet.

Preparing to Juice

- When purchasing fruit and vegetables for juice, look for the freshest, most unblemished produce you can find.
- Before you prepare juice, wash all fruits and vegetables thoroughly under cold running water. Cut away and discard any brown or bruised sections. Remove pits from tree fruit and seeds from grapefruit, lemons, limes, melons, grapes, and apples. Use a brush to scrub away wax, pesticides, and other chemicals from those fruits and vegetables whose skin you will be juicing as well, such as apples and cucumbers.
- Peel citrus fruits and exotic fruits, such as kiwi, papaya, and mango. You can use broccoli stems and celery leaves, but be sure to discard carrot leaves. They contain a toxic substance.
- Buy organic produce if you can find it and afford it.

- Buy fruits and produce in season. The best and freshest fruits, whether organic or not, are available during late spring and summer. If your weight worries revolve around a beach-with-a-bikini-vacation, then you might consider juicing at the time of year when you can get your fill of in-season produce. While today you can obtain a peach at Christmas and a nectarine in February, these fruits certainly will not have the flavor of those grown in season and will also be much more expensive.
- If juice alone doesn't do it for you, see page 49 for a juice and soup menu.

How Much Juice Can I Have?

You can drink as much juice as you like, as often as you want, during the 3-Day Juice Diet. Start out with fruit juice in the morning, followed by a midmorning vegetable juice snack. Lunch, afternoon snack, and dinner can be a combination of fruit and vegetable juices. Included here are several juice recipes, but don't be afraid to improvise. If your favorite fruits or vegetables are not included in any of the recipes, create your own. And if you prefer to start your day with a vegetable—rather than a fruit—juice, switch the juices to suit your taste.

The recipes yield from 1½ to 2½ cups of juice; much depends on the ripeness and liquid content of the produce. You can double or triple the recipes if you wish, and refrigerate the juice you do not drink for a later meal.

EASY ORANGE-PEACH JUICE

2 cups orange juice
2 ripe peaches, peeled and pitted

Combine all ingredients and process until blended, liquefied, and smooth.

CANTALOUPE-BERRY SHAKE

½ ripe cantaloupe, peeled and seeded, cut into
  chunks
½ pint ripe strawberries, hulled
½ cup fresh orange juice

Combine all ingredients and process until blended, liquefied, and smooth.

MANGO-GINGER DELIGHT

1 ripe mango, peeled, fruit cut away from pit
1 cup apple juice
$1/2$ teaspoon shredded fresh ginger

Combine all ingredients and process until blended,
liquefied, and smooth.

SUMMER'S BEST

$1/4$ ripe cantaloupe, peeled, seeded, cut into chunks
3-inch wedge watermelon, seeded, rind removed,
  cut into chunks
2-inch slice honeydew melon, peeled and seeded,
  cut into chunks
2 teaspoons fresh lime juice

Combine all ingredients and process until blended,
liquefied, and smooth.

SPICY APPLE-CARROT JUICE

2 Granny Smith apples, quartered, seeds removed,
   or 1 cup apple juice
4 carrots, green tops removed, cut into chunks, or ½
   cup carrot juice
Pinch cardamom

Combine all ingredients and process until blended,
liquefied, and smooth.

ORANGE, GRAPEFRUIT, AND BANANA JUICE

1 cup orange juice
½ cup grapefruit juice
1 medium banana, peeled, cut into thirds

Combine all ingredients and process until blended,
liquefied, and smooth.

GRAPE-PEAR JUICE

3 cups seedless grapes
1 ripe pear, quartered, seeds removed
1/4 cup apple juice

Combine all ingredients and process until blended,
liquefied, and smooth.

SPINACH, CELERY, AND
APPLE JUICE

1 cup packed spinach leaves
4 celery stalks, cut into chunks
1/2 cup apple juice

Combine all ingredients and process until blended,
liquefied, and smooth.

BROCCOLI, TOMATO, AND SCALLION JUICE

5 broccoli florets
2 tomatoes, quartered
4 scallions, trimmed and quartered

Combine all ingredients and process until blended, liquefied, and smooth.

CUCUMBER, CABBAGE, AND CARROT JUICE

2 small kirby cucumbers, cut into chunks
$1/2$ small head red cabbage, cut into wedges
4 carrots, trimmed, cut into chunks
$1/4$ cup fresh orange juice

Combine all ingredients and process until blended, liquefied, and smooth.

BELL PEPPER, TOMATO, AND ELEPHANT GARLIC JUICE

2 red bell peppers, seeded and quartered
2 ripe tomatoes, quartered
1 clove elephant garlic, sliced

Combine all ingredients and process until blended, liquefied, and smooth.

PARSLEY, CELERY, ASPARAGUS, AND TOMATO JUICE

1/2 cup packed parsley leaves
4 celery stalks, quartered
3 asparagus, tips only
2 whole tomatoes, quartered

Combine all ingredients and process until blended, liquefied, and smooth.

2-DAY ORANGE JUICE AND BANANA DIET FROM BELGIUM

Ginny brought this diet back from Belgium. "It was all everyone was talking about in Brussels," she says. **"You can have only four of these drinks each day. I lost five pounds at the end of the second day, and I never felt hungry."**

This diet is somewhat different from the others in this section: the banana is sliced, not liquefied, which gives you something to chew on, and it is the only juice you will have for two days. Remember, the time limit on this diet is two days.

1 cup orange juice
Juice of 1 lemon
1 tablespoon honey
1 banana, peeled and sliced

Combine orange juice, lemon juice, and honey, and blend thoroughly. Pour into a glass and stir in banana slices.

Serving: 1

3-DAY JUICE AND SOUP DIET

If a juice diet is too limiting for you—even with a variety of juices—you might try another liquid approach: a diet that combines juice and soup with unlimited quantities of each.

DAY ONE

BREAKFAST
  Orange juice

MIDMORNING SNACK
  Citrus Spritzer*

LUNCH
  Clear vegetable broth
  Sparkling water with lime wedge

MIDAFTERNOON SNACK
  Tomato juice

DINNER
  Easy Beet and Cabbage Soup*

LATE-NIGHT SNACK
  Orange, Apple, and Banana Nightcap*

* *Recipes follow for all starred items.*

DAY TWO

BREAKFAST
   Tangerine juice
   Tea with lemon

MIDMORNING SNACK
   Orange-Blueberry Refresher*

LUNCH
   Chicken-vegetable soup (with cubed chicken and
      vegetables)
   Sparkling water with lime wedge

MIDAFTERNOON SNACK
   Beef broth

DINNER
   Tomato Gazpacho*

LATE-NIGHT SNACK
   Apple juice

DAY THREE

BREAKFAST
   Ginger-Spiked Pear-Orange Juice*
   Tea with lemon

MIDMORNING SNACK
   Chicken broth

* Recipes follow for all starred items.

LUNCH
  Cream of carrot soup (made with skim milk)

MIDAFTERNOON SNACK
  Grapefruit juice

DINNER
  Spicy Mushroom Soup with Cilantro*

LATE-NIGHT SNACK
  Pineapple juice

* *Recipes follow for all starred items.*

CITRUS SPRITZER

1/2 cup orange juice
1/4 cup grapefruit juice
1/4 cup sparkling water

Combine all ingredients in a large glass. Mix thoroughly.

Serves: 1

ORANGE, APPLE, AND BANANA NIGHTCAP

1/2 cup orange juice
1/2 cup apple juice
1 small banana, cut into chunks

Combine all ingredients and process until blended, liquefied, and smooth.

Serves: 1

ORANGE-BLUEBERRY REFRESHER

1 cup orange juice
½ cup blueberries

Combine all ingredients and process until blended,
liquefied, and smooth.

Serves: 1

GINGER-SPIKED
PEAR-ORANGE JUICE

Ginger is considered good for everything: According to many doctors, it improves digestion, gives the immune system a boost, and provides energy. All that—and it has a flavor that makes you feel glad you woke up. Try this juice as a morning pick-me-up. It's also great as a late-afternoon snack when your inner clock is running down.

   1 teaspoon shredded fresh ginger
   1 pear, cut into quarters and seeded
   1 cup orange juice

Combine all ingredients and process until blended, liquefied, and smooth.

Serves: 1

EASY BEET AND CABBAGE SOUP

1 cup canned no-fat beef broth
1 cup tomato juice
1 large beet, coarsely shredded
1 carrot, thinly sliced
1/4 small head red cabbage, coarsely shredded
1 onion, thinly sliced
1 garlic clove, minced
2 tablespoons chopped fresh dill
1 tablespoon low-fat sour cream
Salt and freshly ground pepper to taste

1. In a soup pot, combine all ingredients except sour cream and salt and pepper. Cover and bring to a simmer. Cook until vegetables are tender, about 30 minutes.
2. Remove the pot from the heat, stir in sour cream, and season to taste. Stir to combine.

Serves: 3–4

TOMATO GAZPACHO

Gazpacho, a soup and salad combined, is one of the most interesting dishes to come out of Spain. It's a delicious dish at any time and especially when dieting.

INGREDIENTS FOR SOUP

2 ripe tomatoes, coarsely chopped
1 small cucumber, peeled, cut into chunks
1 small onion, quartered
1 small bell pepper, seeded and quartered
1 garlic clove
1 cup tomato juice
1 tablespoon red wine vinegar
2 teaspoons olive oil
1/4 teaspoon cayenne pepper sauce
Salt and freshly ground pepper to taste

GARNISH

1 small cucumber, peeled and diced
2 scallions, thinly sliced
1 small bell pepper, diced

1. Combine all ingredients for soup in a blender or food processor, and process until smooth. Refrigerate until chilled.
2. Serve soup with vegetable garnish on the side.

Serves: 2–3

SPICY MUSHROOM SOUP
WITH CILANTRO

½ pound thinly sliced mushrooms
4 cups canned no-fat beef broth
¼ teaspoon chili powder (or to taste)
2 tablespoons chopped fresh cilantro
Salt and freshly ground pepper to taste

1. Combine mushrooms and broth in a soup pot. Cover and bring to a simmer.
2. Stir in chili powder. Cook 15 to 20 minutes, or until mushrooms are tender.
3. Add cilantro and season to taste.

Serves: 3–4

4

The Protein Approach

I love a protein diet. Meat is one of my favorite foods, and when I go on a diet of all protein and no carbs I'm never hungry, and I don't feel guilty about eating all that marbled steak and lots of bacon slices for breakfast. The last time I went on a protein diet, I stayed on it for four days and lost eight pounds. Boy, was I happy!
— Jean, 28, computer programmer

PROTEIN DIETS: HOW AND WHY THEY WORK

A great jump-start method for dieting and a favorite of many celebrities calls for concentrating on protein-rich foods while cutting down or eliminating carbohydrates. Vegetables and fruits contain carbohydrates, but so do potatoes, pasta, breads, ice cream, cake, and candy. It's the starchy and sweet stuff that will get you in trouble.

Major marathon runners often scarf up giant bowls

of pasta the night before they race. They know that carbohydrates are stored in the body and the calories they provide burn up slowly.

However, if you're not planning to run the New York or Boston marathon, that linguine or baked potato provides calories that remain stored in your body, and if those calories are not burned up, they turn into pounds you really don't want.

"But I always thought it was the sauce on the fettucine that caused me to gain weight," Alicia said. "I thought I could eat all the pasta I wanted."

Sorry, Alicia. The sauce may help, but basically it's the carb-laden pasta that puts weight on—and it can be weight that's hard to lose.

The Big Switch

To lose weight quickly, say a temporary good-bye to most carbohydrates and switch to protein foods: meat, fish, fowl, cheese, eggs, and tofu. Protein works in two ways: As fuel it is used up quickly, and it also acts to burn up fat that is stored in the body. This process, called ketosis, produces ketones (burned off or metabolized fat) which are created as body fat breaks down.

There has been a great deal of discussion, pro and con, about ketosis and whether a high-protein diet, followed for a long period of time, is safe or perhaps dangerous.

The antiketosis side claims that ketones are toxic and can poison the body. On the other hand, doctors who are in favor of a high-protein diet point to research indicating that ketones are not poisonous and are used for fuel by various parts of the body, including the brain and the heart.

Dr. Robert C. Atkins, who has been preaching the cause of a high-protein diet since the 1970s, reiterates his idea in his book *Dr. Atkins' New Diet Revolution,* that a diet almost exclusively of protein not only promotes weight loss but is also a healthful way to eat.

An opposite view is taken by those physicians who state that a long-term high-protein diet can harm the heart, kidneys, and digestive system. They also say that a diet high in animal protein will cause a rise in cholesterol.

The 1980s saw an emphasis on low-fat, high-carbohydrate diets—pasta and whole-grain breads were said to keep you thin and healthy. However, a diet high in starchy carbohydrates is also high in calories, and current thinking recognizes that protein is a fat burner, while carbohydrates stick to the ribs—and everywhere else too.

But What About Cholesterol?

Writing about cholesterol in their book *Protein Power,* Drs. Michael R. Eades and Mary Dan Eades speak out against what they call "cholesterol madness." Cholesterol, they point out, is a building block of the body and produces important and necessary hormones. Cholesterol aids in digestion and is necessary for normal growth and development. It also transports triglycerides through the circulatory system.

While some cholesterol is obtained from food, the majority is manufactured by the body. Lowering cholesterol, say the Eadeses, can be accomplished not by restricting protein but rather by cutting down on carbohydrates.

Some researchers believe that going on a really low cholesterol diet may in fact cause the cells to speed up the manufacture of cholesterol. The Drs. Eadeses endorse a nutritional plan that "relies on food to balance insulin and glycogen," which they say will lower blood cholesterol. Their plan emphasizes protein and includes carbohydrates obtained from vegetables and fruit rather than from breads, pasta, or sweets.

Should I Go on a High-Protein Diet?

The first person to ask is your doctor. If you have diabetes, high blood pressure, high cholesterol, a kidney or liver ailment, or a heart problem, your doctor may give you a firm no. And even if you're in good health, he or she may advise you about certain side effects: Protein acts as a diuretic and can wash potassium out of the system. A loss of potassium can result in fatigue, aching muscles, and dizziness. And, if you are taking certain medications, you may not be permitted to take a potassium supplement.

A high-protein diet also can cause constipation.

"I'm perfectly healthy," Virginia said before she started on the high-protein diet that permitted no carbohydrates. "I know I can be happy eating steak and hamburger and roast beef three times a day."

But by the end of Day 5, Virginia was happy to move on to a modified protein diet that included a small amount of carbohydrates. She yearned for a slice of bread and wanted a salad as well as vegetables.

"Broccoli," she said, "I never knew how much I could miss broccoli."

Each of the high-protein diets that follow (except for the No-Carbohydrate Diet) contains a small amount of carbohydrates. They all offer a fast way to jump-start a diet, and they are appealing because they allow as much protein and fat as you wish.

Suggested menus are included. You may substitute other proteins for the ones mentioned, and you can switch days and meals to suit your own schedule. For example, don't give up on the diet if clams or oysters on the half shell are not available; have smoked fish or a shrimp cocktail instead, or a serving of broiled chicken. You can eat as much protein as you want, and be sure to have lots of liquids.

Meat Without Bones

Perhaps you want to try a high-protein diet, but you don't much care for meat, and you're not wild about fish. A healthy substitute can be protein-rich tofu, called "meat without bones" in Asia. Consider this: 4 ounces of extra-lean ground beef contains 21.1 grams of protein, 19.3 grams of fat, and 265 calories. Tofu, when combined with any broth or stir-fried with a few drops of soy sauce or spicy Szechwan sauce, acquires real flavor, and 4 ounces of tofu contains 12.1 grams of protein, 6.7 grams of fat, and only 110 calories. Tofu—you gotta love it!

Some Dos and Don'ts

A few points to remember if you choose a protein diet:

- You can have unlimited amounts of protein.
- But you can't have any sweets—not even one cookie.
- Limit carb intake to 1 to 2 slices of bread a day, or 1 fruit.
- Even if you choose a high-protein diet that allows some carbohydrates, stay away from starchy vegetables: potatoes, corn, and peas.
- Don't use any sugar in your coffee or tea, though you may use an artificial sweetener, and use either half-and-half or cream—both are much lower in carbs than any type of milk.

How Much Weight Will I Lose?

Some dieters lose 5 pounds on the 5-Day No-Carbohydrate Diet, while others lose 10 or as much as 14 pounds. A lot depends on your metabolism and lifestyle, level of activity, and how much weight you need to lose.

The high-protein diets that include a small amount of carbohydrates work almost as quickly, and 10 pounds in 10 days is not a bad way to go.

And again, don't overdo. In other words, don't follow any jump-start method longer than recommended.

5-DAY NO-CARBOHYDRATE DIET

DAY ONE

BREAKFAST
  Eggs scrambled in butter
  Coffee or tea (with cream, optional)

LUNCH
  Clams on the half shell with lemon
  Chopped steak
  Iced tea

AFTERNOON SNACK
  Wedge of cheese
  Water, any diet soda, including fruit-flavored sparkling
    water (non caloric)

DINNER
  Shrimp cocktail
  Lamb chops
  Water, any diet soda, including fruit-flavored sparkling
    water (non caloric)

DAY TWO

BREAKFAST
  Canadian bacon and fried eggs
  Coffee or tea (with cream, optional)

LUNCH
  Beef broth
  Fillet of sole broiled with butter
  Club soda with lime wedge

AFTERNOON SNACK
  Hamburger (no bun), 2 teaspoons ketchup
  Iced tea with lemon

DINNER
  Smoked trout
  Roast chicken
  Water, any diet soda, including fruit-flavored sparkling
    water (non caloric)

DAY THREE

BREAKFAST
  Smoked salmon
  Cream cheese
  Coffee or tea (with cream, optional)

LUNCH
  Chicken consommé
  Broiled steak
  Water, any diet soda, including fruit-flavored sparkling
    water (non caloric)

AFTERNOON SNACK
  Egg salad
  Water

DINNER
Cocktail frankfurters
Stir-fried shrimp
Club soda or mineral water with lemon

DAY FOUR

BREAKFAST
Cheese omelet
Coffee or tea (with cream, optional)

LUNCH
Oysters on the half shell with lemon
Roast beef
Coffee or tea (with cream, optional)

AFTERNOON SNACK
Cheese wedge with ham slice
Club soda

DINNER
Smoked trout with horseradish sauce
Lamb chops
Water, any diet soda, including fruit-flavored sparkling
water (non caloric)

DAY FIVE

BREAKFAST
Ham and egg omelet
Coffee or tea (with cream, optional)

LUNCH

Chicken consommé

Bacon cheeseburger (no bun)

Any diet soda, including fruit-flavored sparkling water (non caloric)

AFTERNOON SNACK

Assorted nuts

Iced tea

DINNER

Cheddar cheese cubes dipped in hot mustard

Broiled or boiled lobster with melted butter

Club soda or mineral water with lemon or lime wedge

3-DAY ARGENTINE DIET

Argentina is a great beef-raising and beef-eating country. The Argentines like beef so much that many of them eat it three times a day—often paired with eggs. They wash their meals down with the Argentine herbal tea *maté*. *Maté* is not readily available here, so we recommend that you end each meal with your favorite tea, or, if you prefer, coffee.

DAY ONE

BREAKFAST
  Tomato juice
  Hamburger and poached egg
  Tea

LUNCH
  Chicken consommé
  Broiled steak
  Salad with Japanese Rice Wine Vinaigrette*
  Tea or coffee or diet soda

DINNER
  Puchero U.S.A. Style*
  Roasted red pepper
  1 slice rye or pumpernickel bread
  Tea or coffee or diet soda

DAY TWO

BREAKFAST
  Fresh blackberries
  Sliced flank steak topped with poached egg
  Tea

LUNCH
  Asparagus spears vinaigrette
  Corned beef on 1 slice rye bread with mustard
  Arugula and endive salad
  Espresso coffee

* *Recipes follow for all starred items.*

DINNER
Beef consommé with daikon shreds
Roast beef
Green beans
Fresh peach
Tea or diet soda

DAY THREE

BREAKFAST
Tomato juice
Sliced cold roast beef
1 roll
Tea

LUNCH
Chicken consommé
Meat loaf stuffed with hard-cooked eggs
Watercress and radish salad vinaigrette
Tea or coffee

DINNER
Brisket of beef
1 boiled potato
Fresh strawberries
Tea or diet soda

JAPANESE RICE WINE VINAIGRETTE

1 tablespoon lemon juice
2 tablespoons seasoned Japanese rice wine vinegar
4 tablespoons olive oil
1 garlic clove, pressed
Salt and freshly ground pepper to taste

1. Combine lemon juice, vinegar, and olive oil in a bowl or in a jar with a screw top; mix or shake.
2. Add garlic and seasonings; continue mixing until all ingredients are thoroughly blended.

Yield: About ⅓ cup

PUCHERO U.S.A. STYLE

Puchero is a national favorite in Argentina. It's a stew made with beef ribs and a variety of vegetables. The original recipe calls for potatoes, corn, and chick peas, but because those ingredients are heavy on carbohydrates, they won't do on a high-protein diet. Here is a flavorful North American–style Puchero, and the omission of the starchy carbs is no loss.

2 pounds beef short ribs	4 cups beef broth
2 tablespoons olive oil	1 cup tomato sauce
1 medium onion, sliced	1 teaspoon hot pepper
2 garlic cloves, chopped	sauce
2 carrots, sliced	Salt and freshly ground
1 celery stalk, sliced	pepper to taste
1 small bell pepper,	½ pound green beans,
sliced	trimmed

1. Preheat oven to 450 degrees. Place ribs on a shallow baking pan and roast, turning once or twice, until meat is well browned, about 20 minutes.
2. While ribs roast, heat oil in a large skillet. Add onion, garlic, carrots, celery, and bell pepper, and cook over medium heat, stirring occasionally, for 15 minutes. Be careful not to let vegetables burn.

3. Transfer vegetables to a dutch oven or a roaster that has a cover. Place ribs on top of vegetables and add broth, tomato sauce, and hot pepper sauce. Cover and return to oven.

4. Reduce heat to 400 degrees and bake until meat is almost tender. Taste sauce and season. Add green beans and continue cooking until meat is fork tender and green beans are cooked.

Serves: 4

3-DAY EGG AND CHEESE DIET

The great advantage to a jump-start diet based on eggs and cheese is that there are many ways to prepare eggs, and there's a wide variety of cheeses to choose from. This is a good time to experiment with all those cheeses you may have looked at in a cheese shop but have never tasted. Buy small wedges of many different kinds and enjoy them in omelets, melted over ham, and grilled on whole-grain bread or an English muffin. Remember to keep carbohydrates down—you can have as many eggs and as much cheese as you want, but keep the breads and fruits to a minimum for maximum weight loss. The disadvantage to this diet is that while eggs and cheese are high in protein, they are also high in cholesterol. If cholesterol is a concern, this diet is definitely not for you. However, if this diet still has a great deal of appeal despite your health concerns, you might consider preparing egg dishes with egg whites instead of whole eggs. In any case, remember to check with your doctor first.

DAY ONE

BREAKFAST
  Cottage cheese with fresh strawberries
  Coffee or tea (with cream, optional)

LUNCH
 ½ avocado stuffed with egg salad
 Shredded lettuce
 Club soda or mineral water

AFTERNOON SNACK
 Assorted nuts

DINNER
 Egg and mushroom omelet
 Carrot Salad*
 Fresh peach
 Sparkling water or tea

DAY TWO

BREAKFAST
 Swiss cheese omelet
 Coffee or tea (with cream, optional)

LUNCH
 Grilled cheddar cheese on 1 slice whole-grain bread
 Blueberries
 Diet soda

AFTERNOON SNACK
 Tomato juice

Recipes follow for all starred items.

DINNER
Beef consommé
Scrambled eggs with mushrooms
1 slice cantaloupe

DAY THREE

BREAKFAST
1 small orange, sliced
Poached eggs on ½ English muffin with Canadian
    bacon
Coffee or tea (with cream, optional)

LUNCH
Assorted cheese platter: Brie, Gruyère, chevre, etc.,
    with apple slices
Green salad with walnuts vinaigrette
Iced cappuccino

AFTERNOON SNACK
Mixed berries

DINNER
Onion soup
Asparagus and ham omelet
1 slice whole-grain bread
1 fresh nectarine
Sparkling water with lime wedge

CARROT SALAD

3 tablespoons olive oil
1 tablespoon raspberry or balsamic vinegar
1 garlic clove, pressed
$\frac{1}{8}$ teaspoon ground cumin
Salt and freshly ground pepper to taste
3 carrots, grated

1. Combine oil, vinegar, garlic, cumin, salt, and pepper in a bowl or a jar with a screw top. Mix or shake until thoroughly blended.
2. Pour dressing over grated carrots and toss.

Serves: 1–2

10-DAY THINK-FISH DIET

Fish and shellfish are the perfect foods for dieting. Most fish are lower in fat than meat, only a few contain any carbohydrates at all, and fish are loaded with protein. All that—and there is so much variety. If you hate mussels, how about lobster? If the flavor of bluefish and shad is too strong, try white-meat fish: lemon sole, gray sole, Dover sole, and flounder. And then there's salmon—and monkfish, which is called "the poor man's lobster."

With the variety of fish to choose from, and the many excellent ways to prepare fish and shellfish, a 10-Day Think-Fish Diet is easy to follow for you, your family, and friends. For that reason, the recipes that follow serve four.

Cooking Fish

How long should fish be cooked? Many excellent chefs advise cooking fish to a stage of medium rare. When prepared this way, fish is translucent in the center, and the texture is moist and tender.

That's fine from a gourmet point of view, but health professionals advise making sure that fish is thoroughly cooked. Many waters are polluted, and fish can harbor parasites and bacteria that are destroyed only when fish is completely cooked.

Currently, a popular way of cooking fish is by the Canadian rule, which calls for 8 to 10 minutes per inch of thickness. But this is not a hard-and-fast rule. A thin fillet may need less time than a thick chunk of swordfish. Overcooked fish is dry and tasteless, but undercooked fish can be dangerous to the health.

Possibly the best method is to test the fish as it cooks: A fillet or steak should flake when tested with a fork. If you're preparing a whole fish, tug on the dorsal fin—it should come out easily when the fish is fully cooked.

Another advantage of the Think-Fish Diet: You can use butter, oil, and sauces when preparing fish. While a squeeze of lemon may be all some fish need, a coating of sauce can definitely make you feel that you're hardly dieting. But get on the scale 10 days later, and you'll be pleasantly surprised.

DAY ONE

BREAKFAST

   1 slice cantaloupe
   2 slices whole-grain bread, toasted, with butter
   Coffee or tea (with cream, optional)

LUNCH

   Tomato and onion salad vinaigrette
   Smoked salmon with cream cheese
   Sparkling water with lemon or lime wedge

DINNER

   Green salad with blue cheese dressing
   Fillet of Fluke au Poivre*
   Creamed mushrooms
   Fresh strawberries
   Cappuccino

* *Recipes follow for all starred items.*

DAY TWO

BREAKFAST
Cottage cheese
1/2 toasted English muffin with butter
Coffee or tea (with cream, optional)

LUNCH
Lobster salad with sliced cucumbers
Diet soda

DINNER
Beef broth
Chilean Sea Bass Baked with Braised Celery*
1 fresh peach
Sparkling water

DAY THREE

BREAKFAST
Omelet with smoked sturgeon
Coffee or tea (with cream, optional)

LUNCH
Salmon salad
Steamed dandelion greens with lemon and olive oil

DINNER
Steamed broccoli
Broiled shad with lemon butter
1 small bunch grapes
Sparkling water

Recipes follow for all starred items.

DAY FOUR

BREAKFAST
Poached egg and bacon
1 small orange, sliced
Coffee or tea (with cream, optional)

LUNCH
Shrimp salad in small pita bread with lettuce
Iced tea

DINNER
Sautéed Red Snapper*
Steamed spinach with almond slivers
Fresh strawberries
Sparkling water and cranberry juice

DAY FIVE

BREAKFAST
1 slice honeydew melon
½ toasted bagel with cream cheese
Coffee or tea (with cream, optional)

LUNCH
Tomato juice
Curried Tuna and Egg Salad on Lettuce*
Sparkling water (may be fruit flavored, if noncaloric)

DINNER
Asparagus vinaigrette
Spicy Shrimp with Mushrooms and Bell Pepper*

* *Recipes follow for all starred items.*

1 fresh peach
Tea

DAY SIX

BREAKFAST
Scrambled eggs with bacon
Coffee or tea (with cream, optional)

LUNCH
Chicken broth
Sea Scallops Provençal*
Sparkling water (may be fruit flavored if noncaloric)

DINNER
1 slice honeydew melon
Lemon- and Lime-Marinated Swordfish Kebabs*
1 slice whole-grain bread
Iced tea

DAY SEVEN

BREAKFAST
Smoked trout
1 slice whole-grain bread
Coffee or tea (with cream, optional)

LUNCH
Vegetable juice
Sautéed soft-shell crabs
Creamed mushrooms
Sparkling water

Recipes follow for all starred items.

DINNER
  Breaded fillet of sole
  Asparagus
  Blueberries
  Iced tea

DAY EIGHT

BREAKFAST
  1 small orange, sliced
  Pork breakfast sausages sautéed with sliced red bell
    pepper
  Coffee or tea (with cream, optional)

LUNCH
  Shrimp salad
  Hard-cooked eggs
  1 roll
  Iced coffee

DINNER
  Creamy Clam Soup*
  Flounder Wraps with Elephant Garlic*
  1 slice cantaloupe
  Sparkling water with lime wedge

* Recipes follow for all starred items.

DAY NINE

BREAKFAST
 Cottage cheese with diced cucumber and scallions
 1 slice whole-grain bread
 Coffee or tea (with cream, optional)

LUNCH
 Tomato juice
 Shrimp and Shiitake Mushrooms with Jalapeño
   Pepper*
 Fresh strawberries
 Iced tea

DINNER
 Broiled Tuna Steaks with Black Olive Tapenade*
 Sautéed zucchini
 1 slice cantaloupe
 Sparkling water (may be fruit flavored if noncaloric)

DAY TEN

BREAKFAST
 Ham and eggs
 Coffee or tea (with cream, optional)

LUNCH
 Crabmeat-Stuffed Avocado with Cilantro*
 1 roll
 Iced cappuccino

Recipes follow for all starred items.

DINNER
Hot and sour soup with shrimp
Casserole of Monkfish with Spinach*
2 fresh plums
Sparkling water with lime wedge

* Recipes follow for all starred items.

FILLET OF FLUKE AU POIVRE

Steak coated with coarsely ground pepper—steak au poivre—is a familiar dish. This technique also works well with fish fillets.

4 6-ounce fillets of fluke
Coarsely ground peppercorns
2 tablespoons olive oil
1 tablespoon melted butter
2 tablespoons finely chopped flat or Italian parsley
Lemon wedges

1. Coat fish with peppercorns.
2. Heat oil in a large, nonstick skillet until hot.
3. Add fish and cook for about 3 minutes. Turn and sauté on second side until fish is cooked through.
4. Transfer fish to a serving platter or to four plates. Spoon melted butter over fish and garnish with parsley.
5. Serve with lemon wedges.

Serves: 4

CHILEAN SEA BASS BAKED WITH BRAISED CELERY

Chilean sea bass is featured in expensive restaurants. The real name of this fish is Patagonian tooth fish, but as Bill Bowers, the savvy owner of Jake's Fish Market in New York, said, "Who would want to buy this fish if I called it by its right name?"

1 bunch celery, washed and scraped with a
   vegetable peeler to get rid of strings
1 cup chicken broth
1 tablespoon butter
1½ pounds fillets of Chilean sea bass
Mild paprika to taste
Salt and freshly ground pepper to taste

1. Cut each celery stalk in half and place in a large saucepan. Add broth and butter. Cover and cook until celery is almost tender, about 30 minutes.
2. Preheat oven to 375 degrees. Place cooked celery in a nonstick baking pan. Top with fish. Sprinkle paprika on fish and season to taste. Bake for 15 to 20 minutes, or until fish is cooked through.

Serves: 4

SAUTÉED RED SNAPPER

4 6-ounce fillets of red snapper
Salt and freshly ground pepper to taste
1 teaspoon hot red pepper sauce (or to taste)
1 cup unseasoned bread crumbs
2 tablespoons olive oil
1 tablespoon lemon juice
2 tablespoons chopped flat or Italian parsley

1. Season fish with salt, pepper, and hot sauce. Lightly coat fish with bread crumbs.
2. Heat oil in a large, nonstick skillet. Add fish in one layer to skillet and cook until brown on one side. Turn and brown on second side. Add more oil if necessary.
3. When fish is cooked, sprinkle with lemon juice and transfer to a serving platter or four plates. Garnish with parsley.

Serves: 4

CURRIED TUNA AND EGG SALAD
ON LETTUCE

2 7-ounce cans tuna, drained
2 hard-cooked eggs, peeled, coarsely chopped
2 scallions, finely chopped
2 celery stalks, thinly sliced
3–4 tablespoons mayonnaise
$\frac{1}{2}$ teaspoon curry powder (or to taste)
Salt and freshly ground pepper to taste
1 head Boston lettuce

1. Place all ingredients, except lettuce, in a large
 bowl and mix until thoroughly combined.
2. Separate lettuce into leaves and place on a serving platter. Spoon salad into center of platter.

Serves: 4

SPICY SHRIMP WITH MUSHROOMS AND BELL PEPPER

2 tablespoons olive oil
$^3/_4$ pound mushrooms, thinly sliced
$^1/_4$ teaspoon hot pepper flakes (or to taste)
$1^1/_2$ pounds medium shrimp, shelled and deveined
$^1/_8$ teaspoon dried thyme
1 small red bell pepper, diced
Salt and freshly ground pepper to taste

1. Heat 1 tablespoon olive oil in a large, nonstick skillet.
2. Add mushrooms and pepper flakes.
3. Cook over medium heat, stirring occasionally, until liquid from mushrooms has been absorbed.
4. Add remaining 1 tablespoon oil and all other ingredients to skillet, and continue cooking, stirring occasionally, until shrimp are cooked through, 3 to 5 minutes.

Serves: 4

SEA SCALLOPS PROVENÇAL

1½ pounds sea scallops, cut in half crosswise
Salt and freshly ground pepper to taste
1 cup unseasoned bread crumbs
2 tablespoons olive oil
2 garlic cloves, pressed
2 shallots, finely chopped
½ teaspoon *herbes de Provence*
¼ cup dry white wine
1 tablespoon butter

1. Season scallops with salt and pepper and coat lightly with bread crumbs.
2. Heat oil in a large, nonstick skillet.
3. Add garlic, shallots, and *herbes de Provence*. Sauté, stirring, for 3 minutes.
4. Add wine, and cook 1 more minute.
5. Stir in butter.
6. When butter has melted, add scallops to pan. Cook over medium-high heat, stirring occasionally, until scallops are lightly browned, about 3 minutes. Do not overcook.

Serves: 4

LEMON- AND LIME-MARINATED
SWORDFISH KEBABS

1½ pounds swordfish, cut into large cubes
Juice of 1 lemon
Juice of 2 limes
½ teaspoon cumin
Salt and freshly ground pepper to taste
8 large mushroom caps
1 large onion, quartered

1. Place fish in a bowl. Add lemon and lime juice, cumin, and salt and pepper. Toss fish in marinade and refrigerate for 1 hour.
2. Preheat oven to broil, or prepare outdoor grill.
3. Place fish cubes on skewers, alternating with mushroom caps and onion. Reserve any remaining marinade. Place skewers on a broiling pan or grill, and broil, turning to brown evenly. Spoon any remaining marinade over fish as it cooks. Broil for about 15 minutes, or until fish is cooked through.

Serves: 4

CREAMY CLAM SOUP

2 dozen littleneck or cherrystone clams, scrubbed
  and rinsed
1 cup water
1 tablespoon olive oil
1 small onion, finely chopped
2 garlic cloves, pressed
2 celery stalks, thinly sliced
4 cups clam broth or chicken broth, or a
  combination
1 cup half-and-half
Salt and freshly ground pepper to taste

1. Place clams in a soup pot. Add water. Cover and
steam for about 8 minutes, or until shells have
opened. Remove clams from liquid and discard
any clams that have not opened. Reserve clams.
2. Strain cooking liquid and reserve.
3. Rinse soup pot thoroughly. Heat oil in pot and
add onion, garlic, and celery. Cook, stirring occasionally, for 3 minutes.
4. Add reserved cooking liquid and clam juice or
chicken broth to pot. Bring to a simmer and cook
for 5 minutes.
5. Add half-and-half, stirring, until liquid is thoroughly blended. Remove clams from shells and
return clams to pot and continue cooking until
soup is heated through. Season to taste.

Serves: 4

FLOUNDER WRAPS WITH
ELEPHANT GARLIC

Wraps are popular, but rather than using pita bread or a tortilla, try a lettuce wrap—it's great for dieting. An elephant garlic bulb is about the size of a small orange, and each clove is at least five times larger than a regular garlic clove. But although large, elephant garlic is amazingly mild—so mild that it doesn't have to be minced but can be sliced.

4 6-ounce fillets of flounder
2 cloves elephant garlic, thinly sliced
2 tablespoons chopped flat or Italian parsley
Salt and freshly ground pepper to taste
16 large leaves Boston lettuce
1 cup chicken broth

1. Preheat oven to 425 degrees. Cut each flounder fillet in half. Place slices of elephant garlic on each piece of fish. Sprinkle parsley on fish and season with salt and pepper.
2. Wrap each piece of fish in 2 lettuce leaves and place seam side down in a shallow, nonstick baking pan. Pour broth over fish and cover pan with foil. Bake fish about 15 minutes or until cooked through. Transfer fish wraps to a platter and spoon pan juices over fish.

Serves: 4

SHRIMP AND SHIITAKE MUSHROOMS WITH JALAPEÑO PEPPER

$^3/_4$ pound shiitake mushrooms, sliced
1 small jalapeño pepper, seeded and diced (or to taste)
$^1/_2$ cup vegetable broth
$1^1/_2$ pounds medium shrimp, shelled and deveined
Salt and freshly ground pepper to taste
1 tablespoon chopped fresh basil

1. Combine mushrooms, jalapeño pepper, and vegetable broth in a medium saucepan. Cover, and cook over low heat until mushrooms are tender.
2. Add shrimp and cook over medium heat, stirring, until shrimp are done, about 3 minutes. Season to taste and garnish with basil.

Serves: 4

BROILED TUNA STEAKS WITH
BLACK OLIVE TAPENADE

1 8-ounce can small black pitted olives, drained
1 garlic clove
2 tablespoons lemon juice
3 tablespoons olive oil
Pinch cayenne pepper
Salt and freshly ground pepper to taste
4 6-ounce tuna steaks

1. Preheat oven to broil.
2. Place olives, garlic, 1 tablespoon lemon juice, 2
tablespoons oil, and cayenne in a food processor.
Process until ingredients are thoroughly combined. Season to taste. Transfer tapenade to a
serving bowl and reserve.
3. Place fish steaks on a nonstick broiler pan. Season to taste and spoon remaining lemon juice
and olive oil over fish. Broil fish steaks for 5
minutes; turn and broil on other side for an additional 5 minutes, or until fish is cooked
through.
4. Transfer fish to a platter or to individual plates.
Spoon a dollop of tapenade over each fish steak.

Serves: 4

CRABMEAT-STUFFED AVOCADO
WITH CILANTRO

1 pound lump crabmeat, shell and cartilage
  removed
1/2 cup mayonnaise
1/4 cup sour cream
2 celery stalks, finely chopped
2 scallions, finely chopped
2 tablespoons finely chopped fresh cilantro
Salt and freshly ground pepper to taste
2 avocados, halved, pits removed
Sweet paprika for garnish

1. In a bowl combine crabmeat, mayonnaise, sour
   cream, celery, scallions, and cilantro. Mix gently
   until all ingredients are blended. Season to taste.
2. Spoon crabmeat mixture into avocado halves and
   sprinkle with paprika.

Serves: 4

CASSEROLE OF MONKFISH
WITH SPINACH

1 tablespoon olive oil
1 onion, diced
2 garlic cloves, pressed
$^{1}/_{2}$ cup chicken broth
$^{1}/_{2}$ pound spinach, washed, stems removed
Salt and freshly ground pepper to taste
4 6-ounce monkfish fillets

1. Preheat oven to 375 degrees. Heat oil in a large, ovenproof skillet. Add onion and garlic, and sauté, stirring, for 2 minutes. Add chicken broth and spinach. Cover and cook, stirring occasionally, until spinach is wilted, about 10 minutes.

2. Place fish fillets on top of spinach, and place skillet in oven. Cover and bake for about 20 minutes, or until fish is cooked through.

Serves: 4

THREE TIMES TWO

Each of the following three diets—Steak and Salad, Hamburger and Cheese, and Shrimp and Cherry Tomatoes—relies on two basic ingredients. Pick your favorite combination, and focus on those two foods for three days. Remember that no matter how much you love steak, hamburger, or shrimp, you should not stay on these diets longer than three days. However, chances are that after three days you're not going to want to anyway. Menu varieties and suggestions follow.

3-DAY STEAK AND SALAD DIET

DAY ONE

BREAKFAST
  Cottage cheese
  1 slice whole-grain bread, toasted
  Coffee or tea (with cream, optional)

LUNCH
  Broiled filet mignon
  Tomato and onion salad vinaigrette
  Sparkling water with lime wedge

DINNER
  Pan-broiled shell steak
  Tricolor salad of radicchio, arugula, and endive with
    blue cheese dressing
  Diet soda

DAY TWO

BREAKFAST
  Scrambled eggs
  Toasted English muffin with butter
  Coffee or tea (with cream, optional)

LUNCH
  Broiled chopped steak
  Chopped salad: iceberg lettuce, bell pepper, onion,
    cucumber, and radish with Russian dressing
  Sparkling water (may be fruit flavored if noncaloric)

DINNER
Steak kebabs with mushroom caps
Spinach Salad with Japanese Rice Wine Vinaigrette
(see page 70)
Iced tea

DAY THREE

BREAKFAST
Smoked whitefish
1/2 bagel with cream cheese
Coffee or tea (with cream, optional)

LUNCH
Pan-broiled shoulder steak with mustard
Carrot Salad (see page 76)
Espresso coffee

DINNER
Rib steak with sautéed mushrooms
Bibb lettuce, hearts of artichoke, and fennel salad
with Tahini Dressing*
Sparkling water with wedge of lime

* Recipes follow for all starred items.

TAHINI DRESSING

3 tablespoons olive oil
1 tablespoon balsamic vinegar
1 tablespoon tahini
Salt and freshly ground pepper to taste

Combine all ingredients in a bowl or a jar with a screw top. Mix or shake until thoroughly blended.

Yield: About 1/3 cup

3-DAY HAMBURGER AND CHEESE DIET

DAY ONE

BREAKFAST
  1 orange
  Cottage cheese
  Coffee or tea (with cream, optional)

LUNCH
  Cheeseburger (no bun)
  Sliced tomatoes
  Iced tea

DINNER
  Brie cheese on flatbread cracker
  French-style Hamburgers*
  Sautéed mushrooms
  Sparkling water (may be fruit flavored if noncaloric)

DAY TWO

BREAKFAST
  Open grilled Swiss cheese sandwich on 1 slice
    bread
  Coffee or tea (with cream, optional)

LUNCH
  Pizza-style Hamburgers*
  Diet soda

* Recipes follow for all starred items.

DINNER
  Tomato juice
  Hamburger Stroganoff*
  Mascarpone cheese on rye melba crackers
  Sparkling water with lime wedge

DAY THREE

BREAKFAST
  Cheese omelet
  Coffee or tea (with cream, optional)

LUNCH
  Chopped steak with sautéed onions
  Sparkling water (may be fruit flavored if noncaloric)

DINNER
  Onion soup with Swiss cheese
  Grilled Hamburgers Tex-Mex*
  Diet soda

Recipes follow for all starred items.

FRENCH-STYLE HAMBURGERS

When Escoffier, the great French chef, was asked for the secret of his delicious cuisine, he replied, "Butter, butter, and more butter." The French still believe that motto, and yet most French people remain amazingly slim. Here's the buttery way they prepare their hamburgers.

1 pound freshly ground lean sirloin of beef
Pinch cayenne pepper
Salt and freshly ground pepper to taste
1 garlic clove, pressed
3 tablespoons butter

1. Season meat with cayenne and salt and pepper. Add garlic and mix to combine. Divide meat into 4 patties. Place 1 tablespoon butter on a patty and cover with second patty. Pinch meat together so that edges are sealed.

2. Heat remaining butter in a nonstick skillet. When butter is bubbling, add hamburgers. Cook over medium-high heat, turning to brown on both sides, until done to your taste. Be careful not to pierce hamburgers as they cook, or butter will spurt out.

Serves: 2

PIZZA-STYLE HAMBURGERS

1 pound freshly ground lean sirloin of beef
Salt and freshly ground pepper to taste
$\frac{1}{2}$ tablespoon olive oil
2 slices tomato
$\frac{1}{8}$ teaspoon crushed, dried oregano
2 slices mozzarella cheese
1 English muffin, toasted

1. Season meat with salt and pepper and form into two hamburger patties. Heat oil in a nonstick skillet. Place hamburger patties in skillet and cook, turning frequently, until almost done to your taste.
2. Top each patty with a tomato slice. Sprinkle tomato with oregano and top with mozzarella cheese. Continue cooking until cheese melts. Place each patty on one-half English muffin.

Serves: 2

HAMBURGER STROGANOFF

1 pound freshly ground lean sirloin of beef
1/4 cup bread crumbs
1 small onion, finely chopped
1 egg, lightly beaten
Salt and freshly ground pepper to taste
1 tablespoon olive oil
1/2 cup beef broth
3 tablespoons sour cream

1. In a bowl combine meat, bread crumbs, onion, egg, and salt and pepper. Mix well, and form into two hamburger patties.

2. Heat oil in a nonstick skillet. Add hamburger patties and brown on both sides. Remove hamburgers and reserve.

3. Add broth to skillet and bring to a simmer. Stir in sour cream and season to taste. Return hamburgers to skillet and continue cooking, spooning sauce over hamburgers until meat is done to your taste and all ingredients are hot.

Serves: 2

GRILLED HAMBURGERS TEX-MEX

1 pound freshly ground sirloin of beef
1 garlic clove, pressed
$1/4$ teaspoon chili powder (or to taste)
Salt to taste
2 slices Monterey jack cheese with jalapeño pepper

1. Prepare grill, or preheat oven broiler. Combine beef, garlic, chili powder, and salt, and mix well. Divide meat into four hamburger patties. Place 1 cheese slice on a patty and cover with a second patty. Pinch meat together so that the edges are sealed.
2. Place on grill or broiling pan and cook, turning once, until meat is done to your taste.

Serves: 2

3-DAY SHRIMP AND CHERRY TOMATO DIET

This is the diet for shrimp lovers! To follow it for three days, shrimp must be one of your favorite foods, and you've got to love cherry tomatoes. Only at breakfast can you deviate—though there are people who think shrimp is the ideal breakfast food too.

DAY ONE

BREAKFAST
Cottage cheese and 1 slice cantaloupe
Coffee or tea (with cream, optional)

LUNCH
Shrimp salad
1 whole wheat roll
Diet soda

DINNER
Shrimp scampi
Cherry tomatoes and endive salad vinaigrette
Fresh strawberries
Iced tea

DAY TWO

BREAKFAST
1 orange, sliced
1 slice whole-grain bread, toasted, with cream cheese
Coffee or tea (with cream, optional)

LUNCH
Chicken broth
Stir-fried shrimp and Chinese vegetables
Tea

DINNER
Cherry Tomatoes Bruschetta*
Jumbo shrimp sautéed with garlic and red pepper
flakes
Sparkling water (may be fruit flavored if noncaloric)

DAY THREE

BREAKFAST
Poached eggs
2 small slices French baguette
Coffee or tea (with cream, optional)

LUNCH
Spicy Cherry Tomato Salsa*
Shrimp Kilpatrick*
Iced tea

DINNER
Chinese-style Shrimp Salad*
1 fresh peach
Sparkling water with lemon or lime wedge

* Recipes follow for all starred items.

CHERRY TOMATOES BRUSCHETTA

1 pint ripe cherry tomatoes
2 garlic cloves, pressed
Salt and freshly ground pepper to taste
1 tablespoon olive oil

1. Carefully cut each tomato in half and place in a bowl.
2. Add garlic and seasoning. Stir to combine.
3. Add oil and toss gently. Allow tomatoes to rest for ½ hour out of the refrigerator before serving.

Serves: 2–3

SPICY CHERRY TOMATO SALSA

1 pint ripe cherry tomatoes
4 scallions, thinly sliced
2 teaspoons hot pepper sauce (or to taste)
Salt and freshly ground pepper to taste

1. Coarsely chop cherry tomatoes and place in a bowl.
2. Add remaining ingredients and stir to combine. Allow salsa to rest for 1/2 hour out of the refrigerator before serving.

Yield: About 1 1/2 cups

SHRIMP KILPATRICK

3/4 pound large shrimp, cleaned and deveined, tails
  left on
1/4 pound bacon, cut into long, narrow strips
Spicy Cherry Tomato Salsa (see page 111)

1. Preheat oven to broil. Wrap bacon strips around
shrimp and place on a nonstick broiler pan. Broil
shrimp, turning once or twice, until bacon is
brown and crisp and shrimp are cooked through,
about 8 minutes.

2. Serve with Spicy Cherry Tomato Salsa.

Serves: 2

CHINESE-STYLE SHRIMP SALAD

1 pound medium
  shrimp, cooked,
  shelled, and deveined
1/4 pound sugar snap
  peas, trimmed
1/4 cup water chestnuts,
  coarsely chopped
1/4 cup bean sprouts
1/4 cup shredded daikon
  radish
6 cherry tomatoes
1 tablespoon Japanese
  seasoned rice wine
  vinegar

2 tablespoons olive oil
1 tablespoon light soy
  sauce
2 teaspoons sesame oil
1/4 teaspoon hot pepper
  sauce (or to taste)
Salt and freshly ground
  pepper to taste
1 teaspoon sesame seeds

1. Place shrimp, snap peas, water chestnuts, bean
   sprouts, daikon radish, and cherry tomatoes in a
   serving bowl.
2. Combine all remaining ingredients, except for
   sesame seeds in a bowl or screw-top jar and stir
   or shake until thoroughly blended. Spoon dressing over shrimp and toss to combine. Garnish
   with sesame seeds.

Serves: 2–3

3-DAY EGGS EVERY WAY DIET

Eggs are a wonderful high-protein, low-carbohydrate food. They can be prepared in many different ways and can be enjoyed at breakfast, lunch, and dinner. Yet there is a problem in the paradise of eggs: They contain a high amount of cholesterol. As with many other foods, there are opposing views on the benefits of the egg. Doctors who advocate a high-protein diet—and some of them have written very well-received books—are all for eating an abundance of eggs. Others—doctors and nutritionists—look at that elegant ovoid and see high cholesterol leading to heart problems. What should you do if you're considering a diet based mainly on eggs? Check with your doctor. He or she can advise you best on how right an egg diet is for you. As mentioned earlier, an alternative is to eat just the egg whites. And if you do follow this diet, do not stay on it for longer than three days.

DAY ONE

BREAKFAST
  Strawberries
  Cheese omelet
  Coffee or tea (with cream, optional)

LUNCH
  Vegetable broth
  Green pepper and onion omelet

1 slice whole-grain bread
Diet soda

DINNER
Asparagus vinaigrette
Lenke's Egg and Chicken Mousse*
1 fresh peach
Sparkling water (may be fruit flavored if noncaloric)

DAY TWO

BREAKFAST
Smoked salmon omelet
Coffee or tea (with cream, optional)

LUNCH
Eggs Scrambled with Feta Cheese, Shredded Ham,
   and Scallions*
Mixed green salad with Japanese Rice Wine Vinai-
   grette (see page 70)
Iced tea

DINNER
1 slice cantaloupe
Egg and Zucchini Pancake*
Chopped salad vinaigrette
1 small roll
Iced cappuccino

* *Recipes follow for all starred items.*

DAY THREE

BREAKFAST
  Poached eggs and breakfast sausage
  Coffee or tea (with cream, optional)

LUNCH
  Eggs in Tomato Shells*
  2 slices French baguette
  Iced coffee

DINNER
  Almost Avgolemono Soup*
  Scrambled eggs with mushrooms
  1 orange, sliced
  Sparkling water with lime wedge

* Recipes follow for all starred items.

LENKE'S EGG AND CHICKEN MOUSSE

4 hard-cooked eggs, peeled and quartered
1 chicken breast, cooked, skinned and boned, cut
  into cubes
1 medium onion, quartered
2 stalks celery, thinly sliced
4 tablespoons mayonnaise
Salt and freshly ground pepper to taste
1/4 teaspoon sweet paprika, plus more for garnish
2 tablespoons finely chopped flat or Italian parsley
2 cups shredded lettuce

1. This dish can be prepared in a food processor; if
   none is available, use a hand chopper.
2. Place eggs and chicken in processor and process
   until just coarsely chopped. Add onion, celery,
   mayonnaise, and seasonings. Process, turning
   processor on and off and using a spatula to
   scrape down sides of bowl, until all ingredients
   are smooth and blended. Add additional mayonnaise if necessary, and correct seasonings. Stir in
   parsley by hand.
3. Create a bed of lettuce on a serving platter.
   Mound Egg and Chicken Mousse in the center of
   the platter. Garnish with paprika.

Serves: 4

EGGS SCRAMBLED WITH
FETA CHEESE, SHREDDED HAM, AND SCALLIONS

2 tablespoons butter
2 ounces feta cheese, crumbled
2 slices ham, shredded
2 scallions, thinly sliced
4 eggs, beaten, seasoned with salt and freshly
  ground pepper to taste

1. Melt butter in a large, nonstick skillet over medium heat.
2. Add feta cheese and cook, stirring, until cheese has softened.
3. Stir in ham and scallions and cook for 1 minute. Add eggs and continue cooking, stirring, until eggs are just set. Do not let eggs dry out.

Serves: 2

EGG AND ZUCCHINI PANCAKE

1 tablespoon olive oil
3 small zucchini, thinly sliced
Salt and freshly ground pepper to taste
5 eggs, beaten

1. Heat oil in a nonstick skillet.
2. Add zucchini and cook over medium heat until lightly browned, turning occasionally.
3. Add seasoning to eggs, mix to combine, and carefully pour eggs into skillet, covering zucchini evenly.
4. Cook pancake, lifting edges to allow uncooked eggs to flow underneath. Add more oil if necessary.
5. When eggs are just set, slide pancake onto a serving platter. Cut in half and serve.

Serves: 2

EGGS IN TOMATO SHELLS

2 medium, firm tomatoes
Salt and freshly ground pepper to taste
2 teaspoons finely chopped fresh dill
2 teaspoons butter
2 large or jumbo eggs
1 tablespoon grated Romano cheese

1. Preheat oven to 375 degrees. Cut off small slice from top of each tomato. Using a small knife, scoop out tomato pulp, creating a tomato shell. Sprinkle inside of tomatoes with salt, and turn tomatoes upside down. Allow them to drain for 15 minutes. Then turn tomatoes right side up and season with pepper. Add 1 teaspoon dill and 1 teaspoon butter to each tomato.
2. Place tomatoes on a nonstick ovenproof dish. Carefully break egg into each tomato. Bake for 15 to 25 minutes, or until eggs are set. Sprinkle eggs with grated cheese, and place under broiler for 1 minute.

Serves: 2

ALMOST AVGOLEMONO SOUP

Genuine Greek Avgolemono Soup includes either rice or orzo pasta. However, because both those ingredients have too many carbohydrates, we offer a modified recipe that still contains the lovely lemony flavor.

3 cups chicken broth
2 eggs, separated
Juice of 1 lemon
Salt and freshly ground pepper to taste

1. Heat broth in a saucepan and bring to a simmer.
2. While soup is heating, beat egg whites until high and fluffy. Then beat in yolks until the mixture is lemon colored. Beat in lemon juice.
3. Slowly add 1 cup of soup to egg mixture and continue beating. When egg-soup mixture is blended, return the mixture to the pot and simmer until all ingredients are heated through. Do not allow soup to boil or eggs will curdle.

Serves: 2–3

10-DAY SKINNY CHICKEN DIET

Chicken, like fish, is a wonderful food for dieters. Lower in calories than beef and high in protein, chicken can be prepared so many different ways that you'll never be bored with a chicken meal. Neither will your friends or family, which is why the recipes in this section serve four. Because chicken is such a versatile food, this is a 10-day diet. Lunch and dinner call for chicken. No chicken breakfasts are recommended—unless you want to eat leftovers.

Here's a trick to making this diet last for 10 days: Buy a big chicken. Roast or boil it, and use it in a variety of ways over several days.

However, it's possible that while you're dieting you won't feel like doing too much cooking. We polled 40 dieters, and the results came out an amazing 50-50. Twenty dieters wanted to cook more than ever, because they wanted to be near food, while the remaining 20 did their best to stay out of the kitchen. If you are among the latter group, here are ways you can have almost–homecooked chicken dishes. First, find the store that sells the best barbecued or rotisserie chicken. Buy one or more; then, using the cooked chicken as a base, prepare many of the dishes in these menus.

DAY ONE

BREAKFAST
  Cottage cheese
  Coffee or tea (with cream, optional)

LUNCH
  Tomato juice
  Barbecued chicken
  Salad
  Diet soda

DINNER
  Vegetable soup
  Chicken Roasted with Lemon and Garlic*
  Broccoli
  Iced tea

DAY TWO

BREAKFAST
  Strawberries
  Scrambled eggs
  Coffee or tea (with cream, optional)

LUNCH
  Broiled Chicken and Tomato in Pita Pockets*
  Iced cappuccino

DINNER
  Asparagus vinaigrette
  Cold roast chicken
  Apple
  Sparkling water (may be fruit flavored if noncaloric)

Recipes follow for all starred items.

DAY THREE

BREAKFAST
Toasted English muffin with Swiss cheese
Coffee or tea (with cream, optional)

LUNCH
Stir-fried chicken with Chinese vegetables
Tea

DINNER
Breast of Chicken in Avocado Halves*
1 small whole-wheat roll
Diet soda

DAY FOUR

BREAKFAST
1 whole-grain waffle with 1 tablespoon low-calorie jam
Coffee or tea (with cream, optional)

LUNCH
Chicken salad on 1 slice bread
Iced tea

DINNER
Beef broth
Chicken with Broccoli and Red Bell Pepper*
Blueberries
Sparkling water with lime wedge

* *Recipes follow for all starred items.*

DAY FIVE

BREAKFAST
  Grilled cheese sandwich
  Coffee or tea (with cream, optional)

LUNCH
  Broiled chicken
  Tossed green salad
  Iced coffee

DINNER
  1 slice honeydew melon
  Chicken San Francisco Style*
  Sparkling water (may be fruit flavored if noncaloric)

DAY SIX

BREAKFAST
  Bagel with cream cheese
  Coffee or tea (with cream, optional)

LUNCH
  General Tso's chicken
  Tea

DINNER
  Vegetable juice
  Chicken with Pesto Sauce*
  Steamed carrots
  Iced coffee

* *Recipes follow for all starred items.*

DAY SEVEN

BREAKFAST
Cottage cheese
Blackberries
Coffee or tea (with cream, optional)

LUNCH
Chicken cacciatore
Spinach
Espresso

DINNER
Vegetable soup
Chicken in Melon Rings with Spicy Dressing*

DAY EIGHT

BREAKFAST
2 slices whole-grain bread, toasted, with butter
Coffee or tea (with cream, optional)

LUNCH
Chicken soup with chicken pieces
Diet soda

DINNER
Cantaloupe
Curried Chicken Salad*
Sparkling water (may be fruit flavored if noncaloric)

* Recipes follow for all starred items.

DAY NINE

BREAKFAST
Eggs scrambled with scallions
Coffee or tea (with cream, optional)

LUNCH
French-style Fried Chicken*
Iced coffee

DINNER
Tomato and onion salad vinaigrette
Rotisserie chicken
Whole-wheat roll

DAY TEN

BREAKFAST
Strawberries with plain, low-fat yogurt
Coffee or tea (with cream, optional)

LUNCH
Chicken burrito
Diet soda

DINNER
Vegetable juice
Creamy Chicken and Mushrooms Paprika*
Peach
Sparkling water (may be fruit flavored if noncaloric)

Recipes follow for all starred items.

CHICKEN ROASTED WITH LEMON AND GARLIC

1 2½–3-pound chicken, quartered
Salt and freshly ground pepper to taste
Sweet paprika to taste
2 tablespoons olive oil
3 garlic cloves, pressed
½ cup lemon juice
2 tablespoons finely chopped flat or Italian parsley

1. Preheat oven to 400 degrees.
2. Season chicken inside and out with salt and pepper and paprika. Place in a shallow, nonstick baking dish.
3. Combine olive oil, garlic, and lemon juice. Mix well, and spoon over chicken.
4. Roast chicken, turning to brown, until tender and cooked through. Baste frequently with pan juices.
5. Transfer chicken to a serving platter and garnish with parsley.

Serves: 4

BROILED CHICKEN AND TOMATO IN PITA POCKETS

4 thin chicken cutlets (about 1 pound)
2 tablespoons olive oil
1 tablespoon balsamic vinegar
$1/2$ teaspoon hot pepper sauce, or to taste
Salt and freshly ground pepper to taste
4 pita breads
4 plum tomatoes, coarsely chopped

1. Place chicken in a shallow dish. Combine oil, vinegar, hot pepper sauce, salt and pepper, and mix thoroughly. Pour over chicken and refrigerate for 30 minutes, turning chicken in marinade once or twice.
2. Preheat broiler. Remove chicken cutlets from marinade and place on a nonstick broiler pan. Broil chicken, turning once or twice, and adding marinade as chicken cooks. Remove chicken when cooked through and tuck into pita breads. Spoon chopped tomato over chicken and season to taste.

Serves: 4

BREAST OF CHICKEN IN AVOCADO HALVES

1 cooked chicken
2 celery stalks, thinly sliced
1 Granny Smith apple, coarsely chopped
1 small cucumber, peeled and diced
2 tablespoons chopped walnuts
4 tablespoons mayonnaise
Salt and freshly ground pepper to taste
2 avocados, halved, pits discarded
1 head Boston lettuce, separated into leaves

1. Cut chicken into quarters. Reserve drumstick quarters for another meal.
2. Remove skin from chicken breasts, and cube chicken. Place in a bowl, and add celery, apple, cucumber, and walnuts. Add mayonnaise and toss to combine. Season to taste.
3. Spoon chicken salad into avocado halves and place on a bed of lettuce leaves.

Serves: 4

CHICKEN WITH BROCCOLI AND RED BELL PEPPER

1 cooked chicken
1 tablespoon olive oil
1 package frozen broccoli florets, cooked
1 small red bell pepper, thinly sliced
1 garlic clove, pressed
Salt and freshly ground pepper to taste
2 teaspoons lemon juice

1. Remove skin from chicken and discard. Cut meat into large chunks and reserve.
2. Heat oil in a large skillet, and add broccoli, pepper slices, and garlic. Cook, stirring, for 2 minutes. Add chicken to skillet. Season to taste and stir in lemon juice. Sauté until all ingredients are heated through.

Serves: 4

CHICKEN SAN FRANCISCO STYLE

1 cooked chicken
1 cup bamboo shoots
1 cup steamed snow peas
1/4 cup cashew nuts
2 tablespoons olive oil
1 tablespoon Japanese seasoned rice wine vinegar
1/4 teaspoon hot chili oil (or to taste)
1/4 teaspoon Chinese Five Spice powder
2 cups shredded radicchio lettuce

1. Remove skin from chicken and discard. Cut meat into fine shreds.
2. Place chicken, bamboo shoots, snow peas, and nuts in a large bowl.
3. In another bowl, combine olive oil, rice wine vinegar, chili oil, and Five spices powder, and mix until blended.
4. Pour dressing over chicken and toss to combine.
5. Transfer to a serving platter and top with radicchio.

Serves: 4

CHICKEN WITH PESTO SAUCE

2 cooked chicken breasts, boned and skinned
2 cups packed fresh basil leaves
1/3 cup olive oil
3 garlic cloves
2 tablespoons pignoli nuts
2 tablespoons freshly grated Parmesan cheese
Salt and freshly ground pepper to taste
1 head romaine lettuce, torn into bite-size pieces

1. Cut chicken into large chunks and reserve.
2. Place basil in a food processor. Add oil, garlic, nuts, cheese, and salt and pepper. Process until smooth.
3. Spoon pesto over chicken and toss to combine.
4. Serve on a bed of romaine lettuce.

Serves: 4

CHICKEN IN MELON RINGS WITH SPICY DRESSING

1 cantaloupe, peeled and seeded, sliced into 4 rings
2 cups diced, cooked chicken
$1/4$ cup mayonnaise
$1/2$ cup plain, low-fat yogurt
1 small sweet gherkin, finely chopped
1 tablespoon hot salsa

1. Place melon rings on four plates.
2. Spoon chicken into center of rings.
3. In a bowl, combine all other ingredients to make dressing, and mix until blended.
4. Spoon dressing over each serving.

Serves: 4

CURRIED CHICKEN SALAD

1 cooked chicken
2 scallions, thinly sliced
4 red radishes, diced
2 tablespoons mayonnaise
$1/2$ cup sour cream
1 teaspoon curry powder (or to taste)
1 tablespoon fresh cilantro, minced

1. Remove skin from chicken and discard. Cut meat into cubes and place in a large bowl with scallions and radishes.
2. In another bowl, combine mayonnaise, sour cream, and curry powder. Mix thoroughly until blended.
3. Spoon dressing over chicken and toss to combine. Stir in cilantro.

Serves: 4

FRENCH-STYLE FRIED CHICKEN

Salt and freshly ground pepper to taste
1 2½–3-pound chicken, cut into 8 pieces
½ cup all-purpose flour
2 tablespoons olive oil
1 cup chicken broth

1. Preheat oven to 375 degrees. Season chicken, and lightly coat with flour.
2. Heat 1 tablespoon oil in a large, nonstick skillet.
3. Sauté chicken in skillet, turning once or twice, until nicely browned. Transfer chicken pieces to a shallow, ovenproof pan. Spoon remaining oil over chicken and add broth to pan. Roast chicken, turning every 15 minutes, until cooked through, about 45 minutes.

Serves: 4

CREAMY CHICKEN AND MUSHROOMS PAPRIKA

2 tablespoons olive oil
1 medium onion, finely diced
1 garlic clove, pressed
Sweet paprika to taste
2 chicken breasts, skinned and boned, each cut in half
Salt and freshly ground pepper to taste
1 pound mushrooms, thinly sliced
$1/2$ cup sour cream
2 tablespoons chopped flat or Italian parsley

1. Heat oil in a large, nonstick skillet. Add onion and garlic. Sprinkle with paprika, and sauté over medium heat, stirring, until onion is translucent.

2. Add chicken to skillet. Season with paprika, salt and pepper, and cook for 10 minutes, turning chicken to brown both sides.

3. Add mushrooms to skillet. Cover and cook until chicken is cooked through and mushrooms are tender, about 40 minutes.

4. Stir in sour cream and mix to combine. Correct seasoning, heat through, and garnish with parsley before serving.

Serves: 4

5

Cabbage Soup and Other Souper Diets

*Dieting was always a big problem in my life.
That's because when I went on a diet, my husband would complain. First, he doesn't need to
lose any weight, and then he would be irritated
if he ate and I didn't. I found the solution:
soup! My husband likes soup, so I prepare
plenty of it. We both have a soup course and
then he goes on to eat other things while I eat
another bowl of soup. I find I can lose weight
easily if I stick to soup, and he doesn't feel I'm
deserting him at dinnertime.*

—Anneliese, 32, real estate broker

Where does the Cabbage Soup Diet come from? Ask
any dieter who has successfully lost weight on the
diet, and she'll mention the name of one hospital or
another. What you've likely heard is "My friend at
the office told me that she heard it was originally de-
veloped at the Mayo Clinic." Or: "I know it works because my cousin Jeanette lost 15 pounds on it just

before she got married, and she told me that it came from the Cedars of Lebanon Hospital in Hollywood. If it works for those stars, why shouldn't it work for me?"

The Cabbage Soup Diet does work. But does it come from a hospital or any other medical research institution? Not that we were able to discover. It seems to be one of those good dieting ideas that has been passed down over the years through word of mouth because it works so successfully.

As with all the other jump-start ideas, it is not meant to be a long-range plan but rather a way to lose weight quickly.

Is the Cabbage Soup Diet for you? Your doctor has the answer to that question. Tell your doctor—and mean it—that you plan to stay on this diet for only seven days, by which time, if you're anything like Karen, you might have lost as much as 17 pounds.

Not too long ago Karen, an entertainer constantly fighting the battle of the bulge, slimmed down by spending time at a health spa. However, during a cruise to the Caribbean with all those tempting buffets offered on cruise ships, the pounds came right back on.

Though Karen swore that she would never resort to a crash diet again, that cruise changed her mind. Afterward she went on a Cabbage Soup Diet and lost 17 pounds in one week.

Will you do as well as Karen? How about losing 8 to 10 pounds in one week? That's what many Cabbage Soup dieters told us they lost after seven days.

If your doctor gives you the okay for a week of Cabbage Soup dieting, there is still one important question that only you can answer: How do you feel about cabbage soup? You're going to be eating an awful lot of it if you follow this diet. If you hate cabbage and are not keen about soup—no matter how interestingly prepared—this may not be the diet for you. Don't despair. No one diet is right for everyone. Remember, dieting is hard. Don't choose a diet whose ingredients make you turn away in disgust.

If you like soup—except for ones based on cabbage—you might try the 2-Day Broth Diet or the 4-Day Asian Soup Diet. The variety of recipes to choose from presents diets that are crosses between liquid diets and the raw vegetable approach.

Is Cabbage Soup a New Age Miracle?

Sorry to disappoint anyone looking for a miracle, but there is nothing miraculous about cabbage soup. How does it work? Cabbage is loaded with fiber, and fiber is filling, which means you won't feel those pangs of hunger. Fiber also helps keep blood sugar level, and the rapid ups and downs of blood sugar levels are what cause you to reach for sugar-laden foods.

Besides the fiber, cabbage also is low in calories and fat. You can eat lots of cabbage without worrying about gaining weight. As you eat all that filling cabbage soup, your body looks for fuel and finds it in the fat deposits that are stored in your body. And cabbage may be good for you in other ways. It's a member of the cruciferous vegetable family and is thought to be a cancer preventive.

Okay, I'll Eat Nothing But Cabbage Soup for the Next 7 Days

Here's the good news: The Cabbage Soup Diet does permit other foods, but you have to follow a definite regimen. You can have all the cabbage soup you want every day, plus:

ON DAY ONE: Eat all the fruit you want except bananas.

ON DAY TWO: Eat all the vegetables you want, including 1 baked potato with 1 pat of butter.

ON DAY THREE: Eat all the fruit and vegetables you want except for avocado and bananas. Have 1 glass of skim milk or 1 plain nonfat yogurt.

ON DAY FOUR: Eat all the bananas you want. (Well, as many as 7.) Drink up to 6 8-ounce glasses of skim milk, or substitute 1 plain nonfat yogurt for 1 glass of skim milk.

ON DAY FIVE: Eat as much broiled chicken or fish as you want and up to 6 fresh tomatoes.

ON DAY SIX: Eat all the broiled beef, chicken, or fish you want as well as 1 8-ounce glass of skim milk or 1 plain nonfat yogurt.

ON DAY SEVEN: Eat all the vegetables and fruit you want as well as 1 8-ounce glass of skim milk or 1 plain nonfat yogurt.

That's it. Pretty easy to follow. In addition to all the above, you also can drink tea or coffee—no cream or milk—but artificial sweeteners are allowed. And if you want to dress up those vegetables, you can add your favorite nonfat salad dressing.

Wow! This Works So Well I Think I'll Stay on It for Another Week . . .

Remaining on the Cabbage Soup Diet for longer than seven days is an absolute *no*. You can return to it after three months—providing your doctor approves.

7-DAY CABBAGE SOUP DIET

There are many ways to prepare cabbage soup, and we provide some recipes here. You can customize the soups by adding your favorite spices and herbs. Fresh herbs, when available, add a very special flavor to any dish.

BASIC CABBAGE SOUP

$\frac{1}{2}$ head white cabbage, coarsely shredded
3 carrots, sliced
3 onions, sliced
3 scallions, sliced
2 bell peppers, coarsely chopped
4 stalks celery, sliced

1 14-ounce can crushed tomatoes, or 2 tomatoes, diced
$2\frac{1}{2}$ quarts water
Salt and freshly ground pepper to taste
$\frac{3}{4}$ cup uncooked brown rice

1. Combine all ingredients, except rice, in a large soup pot.
2. Bring to a boil. Cover and simmer until vegetables are completely tender and blended together, about $1\frac{1}{2}$ hours.
3. While soup simmers, cook rice and reserve.
4. Stir rice into cooked soup before serving.

Yield: About 3 quarts

OPTIONAL: Substitute 1 quart nonfat beef or chicken broth for 1 quart water.

CHINESE-STYLE HOT AND SOUR CABBAGE SOUP

Basic Cabbage Soup made with nonfat beef broth
  (see page 143)
1 pound mushrooms, thinly sliced
1 tablespoon hot pepper sauce (or to taste)
3 tablespoons Japanese seasoned rice wine vinegar

1. Combine soup and mushrooms in a large soup
  pot, and cook until mushrooms are tender, about
  20 minutes.
2. Add hot pepper sauce and vinegar and simmer
  for an additional 10 minutes.

Yield: About 3 quarts

BORSCHT

1 small head red cabbage, coarsely shredded

3 onions, thinly sliced

10 beets, thinly sliced

1/2 pound green beans, trimmed, snapped in half

4 stalks celery, sliced

4 tomatoes, diced

3 garlic cloves, finely chopped

3 teaspoons lemon juice

1/4 teaspoon crushed dry thyme

Salt and freshly ground pepper to taste

1 quart nonfat beef broth

1 1/2 quarts water

1. Combine all ingredients in a large soup pot.

2. Bring to a boil. Cover and simmer until vegetables are completely tender and blended together, about 1 1/2 hours.

Yield: About 3 quarts

CABBAGE SOUP WITH ESCAROLE AND PARSLEY

1 head white cabbage, coarsely shredded
6 stalks celery, thinly sliced
1 onion, sliced
2 garlic cloves, finely chopped
2 tomatoes, diced
1 quart nonfat chicken broth

1½ quarts water
Salt and freshly ground pepper to taste
1 small head escarole, coarsely shredded
4 tablespoons finely chopped flat or Italian parsley

1. Combine all ingredients, except escarole and parsley, in a large soup pot.
2. Bring to a boil. Cover and simmer until vegetables are completely tender and blended together, about 1½ hours.
3. When soup is cooked, stir in escarole and parsley, and simmer for an additional 5 minutes.

Yield: About 3 quarts

Only Three Quarts of Soup?

"I've read about the Cabbage Soup Diet before," Adele said, "and it always calls for six quarts of soup, but your recipes are for three quarts. How come?"

It's true that many Cabbage Soup Diet recipes prepare six quarts of soup. However, if you get bored easily or are not planning to serve the soup to friends or family, we think three quarts of soup works better. Following a three-quart recipe means that you can prepare different versions of cabbage soup. However, if you wish to prepare six quarts of soup at one time, all you have to do is double the recipes.

Do I Have to Have Cabbage Soup for Breakfast?

Only if you want to. Otherwise, here's what you can have for breakfast:

DAY ONE:	Combination fresh berries
DAY TWO:	Baked potato with 1 pat butter
DAY THREE:	Melon and sliced fresh peaches
DAY FOUR:	Bananas with plain, nonfat yogurt
DAY FIVE:	Broiled chicken with sliced tomato
DAY SIX:	Plain, nonfat yogurt
DAY SEVEN:	Fresh fruit salad

2-DAY BROTH DIET

This is truly a quick liquid approach to jump-starting your diet. The diet requires no cooking; all you do is warm up canned, no-fat broths or reconstitute bouillon cubes. This diet is almost a fast, and though it lasts for only two days, it calls for as much willpower as the water fast. Before you embark on a diet that is so nutritionally limited, talk to your doctor.

What Will I Eat?

You can have as much broth—chicken, beef, or vegetable—as you wish for the two days you're on this diet. You also can have water—plain or sparkling—with a wedge of lemon or lime.

Before and After

Both the preparation and the aftermath of the 2-Day Broth Diet are the same as the instructions for the 1- or 2-Day Water Fast. (See Chapter 1.) Eat lightly both before and after the diet, and though you will see a considerable weight loss after two days, do not continue with the diet past 48 hours.

4-DAY ASIAN SOUP DIET

An interesting way to lose weight quickly is to consume soup from any Asian cuisine. Fond of Chinese hot and sour soup? Japanese miso soup with tofu? How about the Mandarin or Cantonese soups that contain noodles and wonton? All are allowed.

Many restaurants and take-out shops offer Asian soups, and we have included recipes for some of the simpler ones.

Is This Diet for Me?

If you like Asian cooking, you'll enjoy this way of jump-starting your diet. Many of the soups are mini-meals, containing vegetables as well as protein—meat, chicken, fish, shellfish, or tofu. Because these are not clear broths, you may have only one large serving of an Asian soup at each meal. If you wish, you can have an Asian soup for breakfast—see the recipe for congee on page 152. If that doesn't appeal, have tea with lemon.

DAY ONE

BREAKFAST
  Congee* or tea with lemon

* *Recipes follow for all starred items.*

LUNCH

Mushroom Soup with Tofu and Noodles*

DINNER

Cantonese wonton noodle soup

DAY TWO

BREAKFAST
Congee or tea with lemon

LUNCH
Hot and sour soup

DINNER
Beef and Spinach Soup from Korea*

DAY THREE

BREAKFAST
Congee or tea with lemon

LUNCH
Chicken Soup with Coconut Milk from Thailand*

DINNER
Japanese noodle soup with shrimp

Recipes follow for all starred items.

DAY FOUR

BREAKFAST
  Congee or tea with lemon

LUNCH
  Chicken and Lemongrass Soup*

DINNER
  Daikon and Bok Choy Soup with Tofu*

Recipes follow for all starred items.

CONGEE

The Chinese enjoy congee at breakfast. This rice soup may be eaten plain or topped with vegetables, chicken, shrimp, or any leftover. It's the Asian version of our cornflakes with milk.

1/2 cup rice
6 cups water
Salt to taste

Wash rice. Combine rice and water in a heavy saucepan. Bring to a boil, then reduce heat to a simmer. Cover and cook over low heat until rice is like a porridge, about 1 1/2 to 2 hours. Stir rice occasionally to prevent it from sticking to bottom of pan. Add salt to taste.

Serves: 4

VARIATIONS

CONGEE WITH CHICKEN: Add 1/2 chicken breast, skinned, boned, and cubed, after congee has cooked for 1 1/2 hours. Continue cooking until chicken and rice are cooked.

CONGEE WITH VEGETABLES: Add 1 tablespoon shredded fresh ginger, 4 thinly sliced scallions, and 1 cup shredded bok choy after congee has cooked for 1 hour. Continue cooking until vegetables and rice are cooked.

CONGEE WITH SHRIMP: After congee is cooked, add 10 medium shrimp, peeled, deveined, and cut in half. Cook an additional 10 minutes.

MUSHROOM SOUP WITH TOFU AND NOODLES

Tofu, or soy bean curd, has been called by both Buddhists and Taoists "meat without bones." It's rich in protein yet low in fat and calories. Although it's bland when eaten plain, it acquires flavor from the food it's cooked with and adds texture to soups.

3/4 pound mushrooms, thinly sliced
5 cups nonfat chicken broth
1 tablespoon Japanese seasoned rice wine vinegar
1/4 pound thin Chinese noodles or angel hair pasta, cooked al dente
3 ounces tofu, cubed
Salt and freshly ground pepper to taste
4 scallions, thinly sliced

1. Combine mushrooms, broth, and vinegar in a soup pot.
2. Cover and cook over medium heat for 15 to 20 minutes, or until mushrooms are very tender.
3. Remove from heat and stir in noodles and tofu. Return to heat and bring to a simmer. Season to taste.
4. Garnish with scallions before serving.

Serves: 4

BEEF AND SPINACH SOUP
FROM KOREA

2 teaspoons olive oil
2 garlic cloves, minced
3 scallions, thinly sliced
½ pound flank steak, cut diagonally into thin slices
2 teaspoons light soy sauce
5 cups nonfat beef broth
½ pound spinach
Salt and freshly ground pepper to taste

1. Heat oil in a nonstick skillet. Add garlic, scallions, and steak. Cook over medium-high heat, stirring, until meat has lost its red color.
2. Transfer ingredients to a soup pot. Add broth and spinach. Cover and cook for about 10 minutes, or until spinach is tender. Season to taste.

Serves: 4

CHICKEN SOUP WITH COCONUT MILK FROM THAILAND

2 teaspoons olive oil
1 small onion, chopped
1 stalk lemongrass, chopped
1 tablespoon shredded fresh ginger
1/2 teaspoon red pepper flakes (or to taste)
4 cups nonfat chicken broth

1 chicken breast, skinned and boned
1 small tomato, diced
1 tablespoon chopped fresh cilantro
1 cup unsweetened light coconut milk
1/4 pound mushrooms, thinly sliced
Salt and freshly ground pepper to taste

1. Heat oil in a nonstick skillet. Add onion, lemongrass, ginger, and red pepper flakes. Sauté stirring, for 5 minutes. Transfer all ingredients to a soup pot. Add broth and bring to a simmer. Add chicken breast and cook for 10 minutes, or until chicken is cooked through. Remove chicken and cube. Place cubed chicken into a tureen and add tomato and cilantro. Reserve.

2. Strain soup, discarding solids, and return liquid to pot. Add coconut milk and mushrooms, and cook at a simmer for about 15 minutes, or until mushrooms are cooked and liquid is heated through. Season to taste. Pour soup into tureen and serve.

Serves: 4

CHICKEN AND LEMONGRASS SOUP

5 cups nonfat chicken broth
¼ teaspoon hot pepper sauce
1 stalk lemongrass, minced
1 whole chicken breast, skinned, boned, and diced
1 tablespoon shredded fresh ginger
½ teaspoon lemon juice
Salt and freshly ground pepper to taste
1 cup rice, cooked
1 tablespoon chopped fresh cilantro

1. Combine broth, pepper sauce, and lemongrass in a soup pot. Cover and bring to a simmer. Cook for 10 minutes.
2. Add chicken, ginger, and lemon juice.
3. Simmer until chicken is cooked and heated through, about 10 minutes. Season to taste.
4. Spoon rice into bowls, and ladle soup and chicken over rice. Garnish with cilantro.

Serves: 4

DAIKON AND BOK CHOY SOUP
WITH TOFU

4 cups vegetable broth
2 cups shredded bok choy (Chinese cabbage)
1 cup shredded daikon radish
4 ounces tofu, cubed
2 teaspoons light soy sauce
Salt and freshly ground pepper to taste

1. Heat broth in a soup pot to a simmer.
2. Add bok choy and cook until tender, about 3 minutes.
3. Stir in daikon radish, tofu, and soy sauce.
4. Season to taste and heat through.

Serves: 4

6

3-Day Smart Grazing Plan

This is my favorite way of dieting. Running from my office to court, I always snatched a quick bite of food, but my choices weren't too smart—a candy bar, a hot dog. I'm still eating small amounts of food—and I eat all day long—but now I eat foods that help me lose weight. I love smart grazing.

—Melissa, 31, lawyer

Just what is smart grazing? It's a diet that lets you eat eight small meals a day. The emphasis is on protein, with carbohydrates derived mainly from fruits and vegetables and a minimum of starches and sugars.

If you would rather eat eight small meals than three imposing ones, and if you prefer eating at odd hours rather than at those times usually prescribed for breakfast, lunch, and dinner, you may be grazing already. Now all you have to do is to combine your grazing habit with foods that will take pounds off.

What foods can you eat on the grazing plan? You

have so much to choose from that you need never be bored—or hungry. But keep portions small; think in terms of appetizers, starters, and snacks. This is an easy diet to follow if you eat out: Order an appetizer and a salad, or soup and a salad, or soup and an appetizer. The eight minimeals should leave you feeling satisfied but not full or suffering from the sensation that you've overeaten.

All protein foods are allowed: meat (including cold cuts), shellfish, fish (including smoked fish), eggs, cheese, all fowl. Carbohydrates are represented by vegetables and fresh fruit. Limit yourself to one baked potato for the duration of the diet, and avoid starchy vegetables, such as beans (legumes) and corn, and pasta and rice.

While you're on the grazing diet, you may eat a small amount of bread and crackers. But stop yourself from attacking the basket of bread that's placed so invitingly on the table when you sit down at a restaurant. Dr. Herman Tarnower, author of *The Complete Scarsdale Medical Diet*, inveighed against those tempting bread baskets for anyone who is trying to lose weight. Sweet seductions are also out: Cake, ice cream, candy, cookies are *not* foods to graze on.

In the menus that follow we're not typecasting meals as breakfast, lunch, and dinner. Instead, we've numbered the meals from 1 to 8. If you don't hunger for large quantities of food at one time, grazing offers a quick and enjoyable way to lose weight.

DAY ONE

1. Coffee or tea (artificial sweetener and milk or cream, optional)
2. Apple
3. 1 slice toasted whole-grain bread
   Coffee or tea (artificial sweetener and milk or cream, optional)
4. 2 boiled eggs
   Wedge of lettuce with any nonfat salad dressing
5. Diet soda or iced tea or coffee
6. Cup of soup (any kind)
7. Sliced smoked breast of turkey
   Cold asparagus vinaigrette
   Tea
8. Rice cracker and 1 slice of Swiss cheese
   Sparkling water with lime wedge

DAY TWO

1. Grapefruit
2. Coffee or tea (artificial sweetener and milk or cream, optional)
3. ½ bagel with cream cheese
4. Melon with cottage cheese
5. Diet soda
6. Caesar salad
   Iced tea
7. Thinly sliced boiled ham and Brie cheese
   1 French roll
   Iced tea
8. Sliced fresh peach and ½ cup plain lowfat yogurt

DAY THREE

1. Orange
   Coffee or tea (artificial sweetener and milk or cream, optional)
2. 1 hard-cooked egg
3. Strawberries
4. Hamburger (no bun)
   Sautéed mushrooms
   Diet soda
5. Tomato and onion salad vinaigrette
6. Beef broth and 3 saltine crackers
7. Salmon salad on lettuce leaves
8. Baked apple

7

1- or 2-Day Monodiet

A monodiet is based on eating just one food item for one or two days. Two holistic health specialists, Shoshana Katzman and Wendy Shankin-Cohen, authors of *Feeling Light: The Holistic Solution to Permanent Weight Loss and Wellness*, recommend a one-day-a-week monodiet.

They believe that the body needs to be cleansed and detoxified because of toxins that cling to the intestinal system. According to Katzman and Shankin-Cohen, these residual toxins prevent the body from absorbing nutrients properly.

Medical doctors do not use the term "cleanse" except when referring to the complete emptying of the bowels preparatory to internal examinations or surgery, and they generally limit the term "detoxify" to those who suffer from an addiction.

However, both "cleanse" and "detoxify" are in current usage, based on broader definitions supplied by holistic practitioners. Certainly a diet based on one food, eaten as often as wished, for one or, at a maximum, two days does present a rapid way to lose weight and to jump-start a diet.

Katzman and Shankin-Cohen recommend rice for a monodiet—brown rice or brown basmati rice. They also say that a monodiet can be based on any one fruit or vegetable.

A good time to monodiet with fresh fruit juice or fresh fruit is during the summer, when a greater variety of fresh fruit is available.

Some natural health practitioners recommend eating a single food item for one day. Furthermore, monodieting allows you to save time and energy: You don't have to spend much time on food preparation, cooking, or cleanup.

There is also a very practical fact to consider. A monodiet is extremely low in calories. For example, a plain baked potato eaten without the skin provides about 105 calories. Even if you eat three, four, or five potatoes during a one-day monodiet, you will have consumed a maximum of about 500 calories.

Whether you monodiet with plain boiled rice, fruit, or pasta, your intake of calories will be low—and as smart dieters know, calories do count. Naturally, to monodiet successfully and promote weight loss, you must choose food that is low in calories to begin with, and then you must stick to that food for a day or at the most, two. Appetite is definitely diminished when you eat the same food item for the entire time of a diet.

Is a monodiet for you? It might be if you're willing to eat just one food for one or two days. You can have rice—as much as you wish—or any one fruit—peaches, berries, apples, pears, grapes, watermelon—or any one raw vegetable—carrots, bell peppers, celery, and so on.

If you have any health problems or are taking medication, the monodiet may be wrong for you. Even though the diet is of short duration, talk to your doctor before going on it.

One Big Advantage

"The one big plus," says monodieter Lindsay, 37, an ad agency executive, is that "you don't have to think—I mean, no meal planning. Not a lot of food shopping and practically no cooking."

Lindsay has monodieted more than once. She likes the nutty flavor of white basmati rice and cooks up a large pot of it the night before she starts on a monodiet.

"I just warm portions of the rice the next day whenever I get hungry. I cook it only with salt and nothing else. I find that the best time for a monodiet is on the weekend—actually, for me it's the only time. And I pick a weekend when I'm not expecting company or planning to go to any parties or dinners."

Along with her monodiet, Lindsey turns off the phone, collects magazines and books she hasn't had time to read, and spends a day in pajamas, eating rice, reading, and watching old movies on TV.

"I start on Saturday," she says, "and continue until Monday morning. I wake up really feeling better—relaxed, and with energy to face the week. And best of all, I usually lose between five to seven pounds."

If the idea of a monodiet appeals, choose a food that you like—and one that you will be able to live with for one or two days. You can have brown rice, white or brown basmati rice, or jasmine rice (very similar to basmati). Cook a pot of rice the night before you plan to diet and then warm portions as you get hungry.

If rice is not your favorite food, you also can monodiet with one fruit, one vegetable, baked potatoes or with any favorite pasta, cooked al dente, and dressed with nothing but salt and pepper.

We think that a plain baked potato is tastier than plain pasta; two or even one day of plain pasta could discourage any dieter. Baked potatoes are delicious without anything added; and if you don't have a favorite fruit or vegetable we suggest that you stick with either rice or baked potatoes when monodieting.

THE MENU FOR THE MONODIET

1 or 2 days of as much rice as you wish, seasoned to taste

or

1 or 2 days of as many baked potatoes as you wish, seasoned to taste

or

1 or 2 days of any one fruit. You may have as much as you wish.

or

1 or 2 days of any one vegetable, raw or cooked. You may have as much as you wish.

2-DAY ALMOST MONODIET WITH BAKED POTATO

Why do we call this the "Almost Monodiet"? Because we couldn't bear to leave those delicious baked potatoes alone. The following diet may not be quite as cleansing, but it might be easier to follow—but for no longer than two days, please.

DAY ONE

BREAKFAST
Baked potato with 1 tablespoon nonfat yogurt, seasoned to taste
Tea with lemon

LUNCH
Baked potato with 1 teaspoon grated, low-fat Parmesan cheese, seasoned to taste
Diet soda

SNACK
Baked potato mashed with ¼ cup cooked spinach, seasoned to taste
Diet soda or iced tea

DINNER
Baked potato, topped with chopped chives, seasoned to taste
Diet soda or iced tea

DAY TWO

BREAKFAST

Baked potato with 1 tablespoon grated cheddar cheese, seasoned to taste

Tea with lemon

LUNCH

Baked potato mashed with nonfat chicken broth and chopped scallions, seasoned to taste

Diet soda

SNACK

Baked potato topped with 1 tablespoon nonfat yogurt, seasoned to taste

Iced coffee

DINNER

Baked potato with 1 teaspoon minced pickled jalapeño pepper, seasoned to taste

Diet soda

8

Life After Your Jump-Start Diet

Remember the promise you made to yourself before you started jump-starting? You said, "If I could only lose 5 pounds fast"—or maybe you said 10, or 15 pounds— "I'd really start eating right. No more junk food—just let me lose that weight now and I'll be good!"

You Did It!

You accomplished what you set out to do. With discipline and determination you lost those extra pounds that were making you unhappy. You proved to yourself that you can lose weight, and you can become the person you want to be. Now use those same habits of discipline to segue into eating sensibly. The jump-start diet has provided the incentive and self-knowledge; use this newfound understanding of yourself to embark on a nutritionally sound way of eating.

You can lose more weight if you need to, but now you can do it slowly, following a healthful plan that does not limit your choice of foods.

Help Yourself

How can you do this? Here's what you can do to keep on losing weight—and feeling psychologically content:

- Visit a bookstore and browse through the diet section. You're sure to find one or more appealing ideas.
- Join a support group such as Weight Watchers, or start a group of your own. You have friends who are as concerned about weight as you are. Meet once a week to discuss eating problems, and help one another stay on a healthy dieting path.
- Stop eating after 8 P.M. Those late-night suppers can really stay with you. An earlier mealtime gives your body a chance to work off some of those calories.
- Don't stand in front of an open refrigerator, eating a little of this and a little of that. All those little bits of food add up to a lot.
- Drink a glass of delicious, refreshing water the moment you experience even a little hunger pang. Water—plain or sparkling—is filling and oh-so-good for you.
- Buy and wear a belt. You'll feel so good about yourself when you are able to move it one—or even two—notches tighter.

- Don't weigh yourself three times a day. Check your weight at the end of your jump-start diet, and then on a weekly basis when you go on a slow-but-sure diet.
- Remember that all salads are not created equal—especially at restaurants. Avoid those creamy dressings whenever you can.
- Understand that you don't have to clean your plate. Leaving some food is a fine idea.
- Never help yourself to food from someone else's plate because "I hate waste." It's better to waste it than to wear it as extra pounds.
- Never eat when you're not hungry. Eating three meals a day is not preordained. A light snack can be a good substitute for a complete lunch.
- Become active and involved. Exercise and join clubs and organizations that can take your mind away from eating and worrying about your weight.

Supplements

This is the time to look at supplements that can help with weight problems. Among them are:

B vitamins: Help metabolize fat by releasing energy from food. These vitamins also relieve stress—a great help when dieting.

L-carnitine: Stimulates fat metabolism and works within the cells to produce energy. Robert Crayhon, a scientist and the leading expert on L-carnitine, recommends using this micronutrient in tartrate form.

Chromium picolinate: Normalizes blood sugar levels

and works to make insulin produced by the body behave more efficiently. Helps control hunger and cravings for sweets. Also metabolizes fat. This means that you will lose fat (not weight) and gain muscle, resulting in a sexier body

Coenzyme Q-10: According to a study done in Belgium, many overweight people are notably deficient in this nutrient, which helps the body emulsify fat. This could be what you need!

Garcinia cambogia: Extracted from an Asian fruit, it contains hydroxylcitric acid, which is said to inhibit an enzyme that converts carbohydrates into fat. Also controls the appetite.

Ginkgo biloba: Acts as an antioxidant, helps circulation, and provides energy that can substitute for those sugary pick-me-ups you once relied on for a quick energy boost.

Lecithin: An emulsifier. Works within the cells to help fats emulsify. This keeps fat liquid and moving.

St. John's Wort: Used to counteract depression, it can relieve dieting stress.

Are any of these supplements right for you? Much depends on your own medical history. There is no blanket recommendation that is right for everyone, and before you start on any regimen of supplements, talk to your doctor.

Never Give Up

Most people who lose weight do so in fits and starts. Very few manage to keep those pounds off forever. Remember this if you get down on yourself for gaining weight again: You are not alone.

However, if you lost weight once, you know you can do it again. It takes discipline, but rather than berating yourself if you slip, return to a diet. You can go back to a jump-start method, if that's what it takes to give you confidence in your ability to lose weight.

"I went to this fab wedding last month," said Cindy, 23, a physical therapist, "and I ate and ate. Next morning I didn't get on the scale, and I didn't let those diet blues depress me into eating even more. Instead, I went back on the high-protein Argentine Diet that had worked so well for me six months ago, and I got my weight back down in three days."

Keeping spirits high while dieting is important, and here are some activities that can distract you and make you feel better about yourself.

And While Dieting . . .

- *Exercise.* Join a gym, take up jogging, go for a bike ride. And if all of this sounds too active, then walk! The big thing is to keep that body moving. Exercise combined with dieting is a big help in getting weight off and keeping it off.
- *Get interested.* Take dance lessons. Learn to play the piano. Take up tennis or Ping-Pong. Do some-

thing involving. This will help you stop thinking about food.

- *Be a volunteer.* People out there need you. Work with kids who are having trouble learning to read. Take meals to shut-ins. Help out on an environmental project. All this good stuff will give you self-confidence, and that self-confidence will help you break the habit of looking to food for comfort.
- *Be a joiner.* Join the local drama club, book group, gardening club. Concentrating on other things besides weight will make dieting easier. Don't substitute an obsession with food by obsessing with dieting. All obsessions drain away energy you need to be a healthy, whole person.
- *Love yourself.* You're smart, imaginative, funny, intelligent, and talented in many ways. Convince yourself of that, and it will be easier to follow a diet that will help match your physical persona to that beauty within.

BIBLIOGRAPHY

IF YOU WANT TO KNOW MORE ABOUT A HIGH-PROTEIN DIET:

Atkins, Robert C. *Dr. Atkins' New Diet Revolution.* New York: Avon, 1997.

Eades, Michael R., and Mary Dan Eades. *Protein Power.* New York: Bantam, 1998.

INTERESTED IN JUICING:

Calbom, Cherie, and Maureen Keane. *Juicing for Life.* Garden City Park, N.Y.: Avery Publishing Group, Inc., 1992

WANT TO KNOW MORE ABOUT THE HOLISTIC APPROACH:

Katzman, Shoshanna, and Wendy Shankin-Cohen with Melinda Marshall. *Feeling Light: The Holistic Solution to Permanent Weight Loss and Wellness.* New York: Avon, 1998.

FOR INFORMATION ON HEALTH WHILE DIETING:

Diamond, Marilyn, and Donald Burton Schnell. *Fitonics for Life.* New York: Avon, 1996.

Weil, Andrew, M.D. *Spontaneous Healing.* New York: Fawcett Columbine, 1995.

TO LEARN MORE ABOUT SUPPLEMENTS:

Martorano, Joseph, and Carmel Berman Reingold. *Stop Smoking, Stay Skinny.* New York: Avon, 1998.

Mitchell, Deborah. *Natural Medicine for Weight Loss.* New York: Dell, 1998.

FOR HELPFUL TIPS WHILE DIETING:

Danbrot, Margaret. *The New Cabbage Soup Diet.* New York: St. Martin's Press, 1997.

Irons, Diane. *The World's Best-Kept Diet Secrets.* Napersville, Ill.: Sourcebooks, 1998.

BOOKS TO CONSULT FOR SLOW-BUT-STEADY DIETING:

Arnot, Dr. Bob. *Dr. Bob Arnot's Revolutionary Weight Control Program.* New York: Little Brown, 1997.

Aronne, Louis J., M.D. *Weigh Less, Live Longer.* New York: John Wiley & Sons, 1996.

Bricklen, Mark, and Linda Konner. *Prevention's Your Perfect Weight.* Emmaus, Pa.: Rodale Press, 1995.

D'Adamo, Dr. Peter. *Eat Right for Your Type.* New York: G.P. Putnam, 1996.

Fletcher, Anne M., M.S., R.D. *Eating Thin for Life.* Boston: Houghton Mifflin, 1997.

Heller, Dr. Rachael F., and Dr. Richard F. Heller. *Carbohydrate Addict's Diet.* New York: Signet, 1991.

Ornish, Dr. Dean, *Eat More, Weigh Less.* New York: Harperperennial, 1994.

Price, Deirdra, Ph.D. *Healing the Hungry Self.* New York: Penguin, 1996.

Sears, Barry, Ph.D. *Enter the Zone.* New York: Harper-Collins, 1995.

Simon, Dr. Barry, and Dr. Jim Meschino. *Break the Weight Loss Barrier.* New York: Prentice Hall, 1997.

Tarnower, Herman, M.D., and Samm Sinclair Baker. *The Complete Scarsdale Medical Diet.* New York: Bantam Books, 1978.

ADDITIONAL READING MATERIAL:

Baratta, Tommy, and Marylou Baratta. *Cooking for Jack.* New York: Pocket Books, 1996.

Henner, Marilu, with Laura Morton. *Marilu Henner's Total Health Makeover.* New York: HarperCollins, 1998.

Puhn, Adele, M.S., C.N.S. *The 5-Day Miracle Diet.* New York: Ballantine Books, 1996.

Steward, H. Leighton. *Sugar Busters.* New York: Ballantine Books, 1998.

Weil, Andrew, M.D. *8 Weeks to Optimum Health*. New York: Alfred A. Knopf, Inc., 1997.

The Any-Diet Diary. New York: M. Evans and Company, Inc., 1998.

SUPPORT GROUPS

Healthy Solutions for Losing Weight, Structure House
1-800-553-0052

Jenny Craig Personal Weight Management
1-800-815-3669

The Thinking Woman's Weight Loss Program
1-800-448-8106

New York University
Cooperative Care Education Center for Nutrition
1-212-263-7204

Overeaters Anonymous
117 West 26 Street
New York, N.Y. 10011
1-212-206-8621

TOPS (Take Off Pounds Sensibly)
1-800-932-8677

Weight Watchers
1-800-651-6000

Diet Center
1-800-656-3294

ON-LINE HELP

Cyberdiet Health Club
www.cyberdiet.com/new_healthclub_site/health_club/in-dex.html

Diet City: Diet, Nutrition & Healthy Eating Information
www.dietcity.com/

Never Say Diet
www.betterhealth.com/community/nsdiet/tips_art.html